Cholesterol Medicine

&

Muscle pain

Necrotizing Myopathy due to Statin Drugs

By G.L.M.

ISBN: 1543032680
ISBN-13: 978-1543032680

DEDICATION

So many people stepped forward to help us while my wife was hospitalized.

My sister and friends left me dinners in my fridge, attended to our pet, and substituted at the hospital when I needed a break.

Her brother and his wife were there so very often and gave us such special support it's hard to imagine getting through this without them.

I "texted" friends and relation every day, and kept them up-to-date with our daily battle. They were so supportive, interested, and caring.

Many visited to cheer her up, especially our children. A couple took us to the airport while we left our car and belongings behind to be driven home. Friends drove our car home 1200 miles so we could travel comfortably by air to get to our network doctors for follow up care.

The list of many others is too long to go on here, I have privately acknowledged them and their prayers and for being part of our lives. They have all taught me something about life. The only way we will be able to repay these gestures is to promise to pay it forward.

CONTENTS

My wife is recovering from **Necrotizing Myopathy triggered by a statin drug**. This is a very rare affliction. It is more prevalent in women. After over 2 years battling leg cramps, and maintaining this drug therapy on the insistence of her primary physician, the drug attacked her immune system and destroyed her muscles one by one. First the leg muscles, then arms, neck, and throat. The last two muscles in the sequence are the lung and heart. Her normal weight was 150lbs. Her appendages became so swollen, as her immune system turned her muscles to liquid, her weight rose to over 208lbs. The only way to draw blood and administer medicine was through a port in the large artery going to the heart.

The odds of total recovery are about 33%.

Her darkest hours during her **4 months** stay in the Hospital occurred during the 13 days in ICU through the holiday season. During her long stay she endured 3 nose feeding tubes, 4 endoscopies, 2 stomach feeding tubes, 2 muscle biopsies, a bone marrow biopsy, and a bleeding ulcer from harsh medicines. She signed her "X" on a consent form so I could sign her life away. When I asked why a colonoscopy was delayed so long, the reply was, "she was too frail". Shortly after Christmas she whispered she didn't think she could go on, I told her she had turned the corner. She fought a comeback fight that has humbled me deeply.

You may be reading this because you are having difficulty with your cholesterol medicine. Statins are the cholesterol medicines and are being prescribed as frequently as blood pressure medicine and aspirin. There are severe side effects to Statins. Muscle pain should be your first warning.

Not knowing the journey we were about to encounter, I took many notes as we spent the four months in the hospital. I know from my own work experience, the references come in handy when moving forward on decisions. These notes accumulated over the span of my wife's hospital stay. As I looked back on them I realized what a treasure of information I had put together. This **affliction** she endured is rare and there is little information available that would tell the average patient what to expect. **It can be fatal** if it attacks the muscles of the heart and lungs.

I call this an "**AFFLICTION**" because to me it is not a "disease" as the medical professionals refer to it. This is man made devastation **caused by the misuse of modern medicine**. This affliction **can be avoided** with proper supervision of muscle pain, but the message has to get out. We all see the drug company advertisements with more warnings than applicable information. **We** have to be aware of these warnings as much as the **doctors** do. The doctors in their busy schedule may overlook events as they occur during our day-to-day activity. The patient can overlook the symptoms if there is no knowledge. We have to be informed so we can react in time and keep the doctor involved.

There are references here that can save a person future mistakes and discomfort in the recovery process. This is a tough, and rare, situation. Little is known in the medical industry. The professionals are guessing in the race against time, and we are almost helpless to interact.

What you are about to read is an actual account, to the best of my ability, of all the medicines and treatments I was able to witness, and record, during my wife's battle with **NECROTIZING MYOPATHY**. (Necrotizing is Greek for "death", and Myopathy refers to the muscle: "Death to the Muscle")

It is my objective to inform the reader of my wife's experience in order to help them deal with their own problems concerning an adverse affect of CHOLESTEROL MEDICINE (Statin Drugs).

I am avoiding names in all instances in order to be free to share the details on an informative level without offending anyone. To bring actual names into the dialogue would restrict my ability to express the events as I viewed them. I took continuous notes and can now tell this story

Cholesterol is a problem for blood flow and the heart, but we have to pay attention to our own limitations with regard to medication. The medical field is probably on the right tract, but still has a way to go to zero in on the absolute solution with minimal risk. The safety concerns to the individual are still not well publicized.

The older individuals that are coming to the hospital with this affliction are just now showing the results of a drug therapy that they started over a quarter century ago. This is on the rise. It doesn't have to be. **It may be possible we are developing intolerance to the drug over the long period of time.** We have to know when to make an adjustment before falling victim to this terrible result. I have read articles that suggest women over 75 should not continue this therapy, and they are 10 times more likely than men to develop this affliction.

As you read on you will be better informed of the journey involved in this devastating affliction. If it has happened to you, you will be ready for things that may come along the way and can avoid them or better control them.

Hopefully, you are not reading this because you are already at the worst level. It would be better to catch this problem at the early stages. **If you have muscle pain, I urge you to start your corrections now.**

Take the journey with me now as we travel through an experience no one should ever have to endure.

Chapter One

THE BEGINNING OF A LONG JOURNEY

During the years before everything backfired my wife was seeing her primary doctor for her general care. One of her concerns was a history of heart illness in the family. Although her mother lived to be 99, her father died of a heart attack at 61. His father and brother also died of heart attacks as far as she was told.

She had a fear of the genetics that might put her in danger, and consulted with her doctor along these lines. Her cholesterol numbers were under 300, at around 280. While these numbers were high, there are ways of controlling them, avoiding clogged arteries and possible heart attack. He prescribed a generic statin drug to lower cholesterol.

She maintained this statin drug therapy for over

12 years. In the last two years of taking the drug she started developing severe leg cramps.

I will point out my own experience here. My own doctor switched my brand of cholesterol medicine at the mere mention of leg cramps.

In my wife's case her doctor told her to maintain the medicine and the dosage of 40 mg. In the early years she was taking 10mg per day. Over time the doctor kept increasing the dosage until it reached 40mg per day for well over the last 2 years.

The last two years, just before the hospitalization, I spent many nights getting up during the wee hours helping stretch her upper thigh muscles. This would help until I let go. It took a lot of strength and I couldn't maintain my strength long enough to make the cramp go away. Other nights she would get up with foot cramps which seemed to occur with just the rubbing of her toes on the sheets.

Despite talking to the doctor about this, he insisted she stay on the statins she was taking. He told her to drink more water, and urged her to seek out quinine water. (The amount of quinine that would be needed could not be consumed in this product). The FDA does not recommend quinine treatment anymore. This was used during WWII to battle Malaria.

The year our problem occurred we were traveling to warmer weather for the winter.

On October 9, 2015 she saw a local dermatologist for a rash on her cheek. She was given an ointment to apply.

On her 75th birthday, November 13, about 2 weeks after setting up house in our southern address, she woke to a swelling around the jaw area of her face. She came into our living room that morning and asked if her face looked swollen. It appeared puffed on the right side of her jaw.

It might be good to note here that she also had a red irritated right cheek. The cheek appeared to be surface capillaries that may have been a indicator of the body's fight from within. This was the rash area she had been treating. She was also experiencing progressive weakness. These were very confusing symptoms never experienced before.

We visited the **local clinic** right away that Friday morning. After some hassle about out of network coverage on our health insurance, we were cleared to enter for an examination. Our insurance company recommended this clinic. We insisted they call their billing department. When they did they were surprised to find our carrier was registered with them. **It took that extra effort to get through the door.**

The attending physician determined that the swelling was due to the "rash" and **a possible salivary tract infection**. He prescribed Amoxicillin/Clavulanic acid(a common antibiotic). We were sent home to follow directions of a daily dose for 10 days.

After a few days, there didn't appear to be any improvement. With concern that the condition was worsening on November 18th we went to the emergency room of the local hospital to seek out a better diagnosis. She got a CT scan of her upper jaw and neck area and blood drawn for testing. They came to **the same conclusion** as diagnosed at the clinic. They prescribed a stronger antibiotic

Clindamycin. Once again we returned home to anticipate the results.

Since the initial visit on November 13, there was also the continuing weakness occurring in her muscles.

On November 20th I had a regular check up scheduled with my heart doctor. During that visit I expressed my concern for my wife's health. With my explanation he instructed me to return on Monday with her if she wasn't getting better. He said he would see her without an appointment.

We spent that agonizing weekend with no apparent improvement on her condition. In fact, she was getting worse. The next Monday morning, the 23rd, we were at my heart doctor's office for his help and evaluation. We were initially put off by the receptionist and office manager, because we were not following normal procedure for appointment. However, after some explanation and a phone call to the doctor we were escorted into a waiting room. The doctor graciously gave us his time in-between his scheduled appointments for the day. He thoroughly examined her, including blood pressure and heart. He promised to get us to the doctors we needed, and soon.

By this time the swelling on her face advanced to both sides and gave the appearance of weight gain. On that same Monday afternoon, the 23rd, we received a phone call from my heart doctor's office. They had arranged for my wife to see a dermatologist that very afternoon. We arrived early and filled out their health history questionnaire. Our session with this doctor came with a new diagnosis. **It was determined that the rash on the cheek needed a stronger antibiotic** that would be sure to work. He said the swelling would subside as well. He has seen this before. We went to the drugstore on the way home to pick up SMZ-TMP SS tab (another antibiotic).

The following morning, November 24th, we received another call from my heart doctor. He had made contact with a primary physician for us. We called the new doctor's office and they made room for us right away that Tuesday afternoon. We once again were sure to be early and filled out the necessary lengthy paperwork while my wife labored in her weakened condition.

The doctors were covered by our Health Insurance provisions for out of network care. This doctor, with respect for _my_ doctor's wishes, gave my wife a thorough examination. **He questioned the diagnosis from the dermatologist, but was respectful of his opinion.** This doctor was interested in a full blood work-up. The weigh-in during that visit was 156lbs., blood pressure was 152/80..

On the trip home that afternoon we located a clinic along the way. We were left with just 15 minutes to spare, to get into the Lab for the blood work needed, before they closed. The hours posted on the door indicated it would close at 4pm. I went in first and asked if they would take us at this close time to closing. They said they couldn't and I would have to come back tomorrow. Then the clerk said she was kidding and would be glad to take us now. Time seemed to be of the essence as my wife continued to lose strength. The blood draw was done and within 20 minutes or so, we were on our way home.

Early the next morning, November 25th, we received a phone call from the primary doctor's office instructing us to **get to a hospital right away because the sodium count in the blood test was 113.** Not knowing what that level indicated we followed the instructions and immediately dressed for the trip to the emergency room at the Regional Hospital. She was examined at 10:30AM, and given an EKG. Blood was drawn and an IV was started. By 3:30PM she was assigned to an ICU room for close monitoring. They would start an IV sodium drip to slowly increase the count over the next 3 days. **We learned that if the sodium count had gone any lower she risked going into a coma.**

At 4:50PM another EKG was performed and at 6:30PM the new sodium count was 117. With the muscle weakness came a bladder problem. The sonogram showed 694ml of urine, 300ml is considered normal. They tried a bedpan first but had to resort to catheterization. An infectious disease doctor prescribed Clindomycin intravenously to control possible uterine infection from the catheter.

At 11:00AM on November 26, blood pressure was 143/64. She was given oral oxycodone for pain. Also an IV was started to promote urination to relieve the swelling from perceived water retention. At 12 noon blood pressure reading was 138/63. They couldn't find a vein to draw blood due to the swelling. At 12:45PM another attendant came in and was successful in getting a blood sample from her arm. The catheter remained for the bladder. At 1:30PM blood pressure was 141/60. She was able to consume some thanksgiving dinner comprised of Turkey, cranberries, sweet potato, etc. A stronger dose of sodium was started with the current count at 118. The blood pressure reading taken at 2:12PM was 131/65. A new antibiotic was added through the IV at 2:42PM.

She was taken for an x-ray for back pain. The bed and all monitors went with her. She had to stand up for this x-ray. Although she was horribly weak by this time, she managed to stand for the procedure despite being somewhat lightheaded during the term. She returned to her ICU room at 3:05PM.

4:12PM blood pressure 128/60. She sounded slow and weaker when speaking. This might be due to a lack of sleep the night before, and she had many visitors during this day which could have dragged her energy down. The recent sodium count came back at 127 and holding. Temperature was taken and recorded at 97.6°. An ENT doctor checked the rash on her face and decided it is not a salivary gland infection. He set up an order for a sonogram of the neck area and the rash.

8:00PM blood pressure 104/52, Sodium count was reported at 118. The difficulty of regulating this number was becoming more confusing. We were told the rise had to be controlled. If it went up too fast there were other complications that could result. The sonogram that was ordered was scheduled for the next day.

November 27th, at 10:30AM blood pressure is 111/54. The sonogram is going to be very soon. Sodium count is now 120 and they determined that the urine is normal. Now they want to get more aggressive on pushing the sodium count up. The rash on the face seems to be drying up. They ordered a CAT scan for the chest and one for the stomach. The main objective is to find a cause for the swelling.

At 2:51PM someone tried to find a vein to draw blood. This was unsuccessful because of the swelling. Consideration of a "PICC" line was thought to be a bad option at this time.

A dietitian came in at 3:02PM to discuss a soft diet to help her during this developing swallowing difficulty.

A very informative visit came from a Rheumatologist at 3:10PM. He was exploring various diagnoses. His first option was Dermatomyositis. This, as he explained, is when Enzymes attack muscles and skin. A biopsy of the quadriceps muscle would be required.

At 3:45PM a doctor came to put a central line in her neck, **since the swelling of her appendages was so severe it was difficult to find a vein** each time they needed to draw blood for tests. This is a semi-permanent line in which they can take blood samples and administer IV medicine as needed without needing to prod for a vein. We were told that as the swelling grows it puts pressure on the vein and constricts the size of the vein making it more difficult to access. The central line overcomes that obstacle.

At 3:46 the Rheumatologist was leaving and said that the enzyme levels report could come back negative and they can get her back to normal, but we will have to wait and see.

The central line in her neck was completed at 4:15PM. An x-ray was taken to be sure it was in the proper place. Now they can readily draw blood samples for future testing. The x-ray determined insertion was correct. It looks like a one inch patch on the right side of her neck just below the jaw bone.

At 5:00pm she was taken for the CAT scan of her chest and abdomen. I took a break at this time. At 8:00pm they changed the bedding, and informed me the last sodium count was 120. Not knowing what to expect this seemed to be encouraging news. It was up 7 points from where we started.

The morning of November 28, at 10:00am the

sodium count was reported at 129. The primary doctor visited at 11:00am and said he was going to try to keep her in ICU for a better watch. He said the biopsy they are looking to perform will have to be done on Tuesday December 1. They were hoping to do it on Monday, but the doctor that performs this operation is not available to the hospital until then. The computers went down for 2 days over the Thanksgiving weekend to add to our frustration. Although the nurses and doctors attended to her needs, the access to thorough records was not there.

At 1:00pm she said this lunch hour was the first time her stomach growled but **she didn't have the strength to feed herself**. She received a few visitors over the course of the afternoon. I stayed to feed her at 5:00pm.

At 8:00pm the nurse removed my wife's socks and the elastic bands around her lower legs to give her skin a chance to breathe. The elastic is to reduce the chance of blood clots. They will put them back on before she goes to sleep. I also took the wedding rings off her finger at the suggestion of the nurse before swelling got worse. It was already bad timing. I had to use a soapy solution to get the job done.

They stopped the intravenous feeding and will restart it when the new medicine dosage arrives. Unfortunately they wanted to wait for the computers to come back on line. In the meantime I am wondering how far this illness will progress while they wait. It doesn't seem right. I am thinking about all those times I heard it was better to catch a problem early.

The morning of November 29 they took a lot of blood samples. We are expecting a new sodium count soon. They said they are trying to address the swelling. She got a bath session in the bed at 6:00am. She complained her mouth was dry. It was assumed this was from the diuretic. She also said she had a rotten night's sleep.

The kidney specialist said he wants to explore the possibility of Myasthenia Gravis. I looked it up and felt it didn't fit. It was similar to Guillain-Barre disease. The head nurse said they had eliminated these possibilities. About this time the sodium count report came back at 127. The primary doctor said they are focusing on the results they will get from the biopsy on Tuesday. He said she tested positive for Rheumatoid arthritis which is inflammatory, but the early tests are negative for autoimmune problems. We haven't had the muscle biopsy done yet.

On November 30 the swelling on the face seems to be down. A doctor came in that morning to say they are testing for mixed connective tissue disease. At 11:00am they started another IV for sodium. At 1:00pm the doctor for the biopsy stopped by to say the procedure will be at 8:30am Tuesday morning and that it is a small incision. When it is done they sew it up and use super glue and the healing will take 2 to 6 weeks. He said some people have played golf the day after. That won't happen this time of course. Steroids will be administered after the biopsy. **They don't want to give steroids right away because they fear a false reading from the biopsy.** The steroids should take the swelling down, we were told. The muscle tissue sample will be driven to a lab in children's hospital, since they have no lab at this regional hospital to obtain the proper results.

At 1:15pm the primary doctor came by to say he wants to get the sodium up so the biopsy will not be delayed. Then steroids will follow. He still cannot give a firm diagnosis until after they see the biopsy results. By this time we have had two resident nurses who say this primary doctor is "the best". The nurse is giving her 80mg of Lasix diuretic IV to increase urine output and hopefully reduce the swelling due to fluid retention. By 2:15 the infectious disease doctor declared she did not need any more antibiotics.

I arrived early on Tuesday December 1st. I knew she was having the biopsy procedure early. At 7:50am they wheeled her out of the room for the biopsy procedure. At 8:24am the tally board showed her "in holding" as I sat in the waiting room. At 10:45 she was returned to her room in ICU where they took more blood samples. **She mentioned her arms swelled up overnight.** They are down now, and the facial swelling seems to be subsiding also. At 1:30pm the primary doctor says that we may have some preliminary knowledge from the biopsy tomorrow or the next day. They do some examination here at the hospital. He also said it sometimes takes up to two weeks to get a firm answer from the lab they send it out to. In the meantime, we will be starting her on steroids and by tomorrow we will move her out of ICU if all is well.

They started the steroids by IV at 5:15pm. At 8:00pm the rheumatologist said he was thinking the muscle is dropping sodium. The muscle count is 3000, down from 7000. I was not sure what that means. They give information quickly. It comes as a surprise since this is all new to us. I probably should have asked more questions to get a better education on her situation. I learned much later that this is the CK count which indicates the level of the muscle damage. A normal count is under 100.

Her hands swelled again. They will be exploring the other two diseases depending on the outcome of the biopsy. The doctor said after the steroids start working they will send her to physical therapy if she feels up to it. This sounds very promising.

On the morning of Wednesday December 2, I arrived to find the steroids are working and **she feels much better**. She was sitting up eating breakfast and in good spirits. I was overwhelmed with hope. Tears welled up in my eyes as I watched her. She asked me what was wrong. I told her the tears were for the joy I was feeling, thinking we turned the corner on a mysterious future. Her vitals are great. The nurse thinks we are getting her out of ICU and into a regular private room sometime later today or first thing in the morning. The kidney doctor told her the sodium count is 134 and the swelling is down because of the lasix diuretic. I am cautiously thinking things are going to be okay.

At 1:45pm the primary doctor said the steroids are taking care of everything and there is no definitive diagnosis yet. He thinks they will move her out of ICU either tonight or tomorrow morning. She will be on intravenous steroids and tomorrow they will start on oral pill steroids.

They have ruled out allergy and thyroid problems. If she improves and the sodium count holds (134) they will release her and follow up out of the hospital. Great news!

At 2:00pm they came in with a wheelchair to move her to a private room on the second floor. At 4:45pm the primary doctor said **preliminary results** from the in house lab show a muscle that hasn't been used enough compared to what it should look like for a person as active as she is. This is causing him concern. He is also going to confide in a doctor for her throat and nasal issues.

Thursday, 9:35am, December 3rd her blood pressure is 127/60, but she seems to have regressed. Her lungs were checked and they have her sitting up. **The swelling returned, and she is very weak**. They have restricted the fluid intake to 1200mg per day. **Some slurred speech is becoming noticeable**. This is getting scary. At 10:30am she finally went to the bathroom after a week. The nurse checked the central line at

11:55am and gave her Prednisone (steroid). At 2:00pm her blood pressure was high because they took her off some medication. They put her on Norvasc (Amiodipine) which is used alone or in combination with other medications to treat high blood pressure and chest pain (angina). Amiodipine is in a class of medications called calcium channel blockers. It lowers blood pressure by relaxing the blood vessels so the heart does not have to pump as hard.

At 5:30pm a neurologist came in and had her do exercises to determine her alertness. She had to follow his finger with her eyes, and various similar exercises. The conclusion is the problem is still in the muscle area and the original target diagnosis is still the path to take. The nurse leader checked in at 5:45pm to see if her needs were being attended to.

At 6:20pm the rheumatologist said they are perplexed. They thought the steroids would have her feeling great by today. They are now looking at a possible diagnosis of dermatomyositis or polymyositis. At 6:45pm the sodium count is now 127.

Friday morning, 10:00am, December 4th, **she seems worse.** She is still not responding to steroid medication. The doctors made special visits last night to reassess. She is still weak and swollen. A new antibiotic is due to be administered at noon. At 1:00pm she asked for pain medication. She said she was a 10 on the scale of "1 to 10". She received 3 pills. The primary doctor stopped in to say he will check with the rheumatologist for the possible use of intravenous immunoglobulin. We are told this is the given treatment for this category of autoimmune illness. It helps the body repair itself.

I mentioned Lime Disease as a possibility. He said they could run tests. At 1:30pm the dietitian said they will giver her Nepro (a food supplement nutritional drink) to get the protein, and yogurt for food substance. This will keep the liquid consumption down so we don't contribute to the swelling problem. At 2:15pm she received a call from her sister saying her father's mother had TB, just as a piece of information.

At 4:00pm the doctor said steroids are the treatment for the suspected diagnosis of dermatomyositis. Any diagnosis concerning myopathy would get this kind of treatment also. The nurse just came in and gave her a larger dose of steroids. **They are trying 80mg.**

December 5th, 10:30am the nurse is setting up the next dose of steroids. They will administer something in the IV to take care of the **nausea**. She feels lousy. The sodium count is 125. The Rheumatologist says the muscle enzyme levels are down from 1500 to 700. This is good. **He suspects statin damage**. He says the steroids should have worked by now. He will refer us to a practicing University specialist. **He also added that they scanned her "head to toe" for cancer which appeared negative**.

At 1:25pm a team doctor showed up to say they are still not sure what to diagnose. The primary doctor will be back Monday to discuss what is next.

At 3:55pm the nurse leader stopped to check on

service. 7:05pm vitals were 115/60. At 8:30 she got a pain pill, the Lasix, and a slow release of steroids IV. The dressing on the neck central line has to be replaced for cleanliness.

December 6th a new attending doctor admitted he was substituting for our primary doctor and not familiar with her case. He said he worked with the primary doctor assigned to her case. We didn't ask him much because he obviously didn't do much homework to be of any help. He didn't seem to have our interest at heart. He didn't seem to care either. It is awful having to wait for answers. We have an enterologist consultation tomorrow to make sure there is no blockage or problem with the stomach. She needs to be able to eat. We are surprised to have the enterologist show up today. He examined her. He found her stomach was painful to the touch. An Endoscopy was ordered for tomorrow. They also added medicine for the yeast infection in her throat. Her mouth and throat have been so dry. She has thrush. She was scraping little dry pyramids from the back of her tongue. They looked like miniature chocolate drops, pointy, and about 1/16-1/8" in diameter. The nurse suggested I purchase Biotene Dry Mouth Moisturizing Liquid spray. It seemed odd to me, that a hospital would not have this item for the patient's comfort. (This will become her constant demand item throughout her stay.)

She is receiving IV antibiotics added by an attending doctor. At 4:53pm she is given Lovenox to prevent blood clots.

December 7th she expressed more pain. She has little urine output. She's alert and agitated. They scheduled a CT scan to see what else might be happening. The head nurse requested a Rapid Response Team to evaluate her care, since so many things seem to be regressing. I felt panicky over that news. I was not sure what was going on. I started fearing the worst. The term "Rapid Response" tells me something might happen quickly and they have to be ready. Actually, they were an evaluation team that is called in to oversee the treatment and be sure she is getting it in a timely manner. This was a very special case. I was not handling the information well.

Her heart rate increased to 120bpm. We were told the CT scan was scheduled for abdominal examination. At 11:30am she was taken for an endoscopy to check the stomach for the "burning" issue. I waited in the waiting room. At 12:00 they brought her back without the procedure being done. **They did not want to risk anesthesia in her weakened condition**. 1:30pm the infectious disease doctor ordered Diflucan to combat the throat infection that is resulting in "thrush".

2:00pm more steroids were administered. We were told **it is for muscle and breathing**. 2:10pm drawing more blood samples. About 3:00pm the doctors came in to discuss treatment with IVIG (Intravenous Immunoglobulin) which puts a great amount of platelets and antibodies into the blood stream to help fight off the attack of the immune system. They also told us she was accepted at the General Hospital, but we would be on standby waiting for the availability of a bed. This news was the result of previous discussions with the doctors as they labored through their diagnosis. They suggested that a bigger hospital might have the experts we needed to get the care she needed. I was not sure if they were just passing the responsibility or guiding us to the better answers. After some time I started to think this would be a good option.

December 8th, 8:30am the nurse said she needs a blood transfusion because her hemoglobin has dropped to 7.2. Anything under 7 is considered dangerous. 11-15 count is considered normal. At 9:10am they are taking blood samples to match as closely as possible to a whole blood donor. The speech therapist came by at 9:30am to assess her throat. Antacids were given at 11:30am for her burning stomach. Sugar count was horribly high at 440, at a 12:15pm check. 12:45pm she got more Diflucane for the stomach. 1:00PM was the start of the IV blood transfusion, type A+. They have to stand by for the first 15 minutes to see if there is any adverse reaction by the patient to this foreign product. This is standard procedure, since it isn't her own blood. The risk is small, but the caution is taken. This was a bit unnerving. At 1:30pm the reported sugar count is 455. The nurse was trying to get answers for this surge. The primary doctor came by at 1:45pm to discuss the high sugar reading. He advised us that the sugar is pushed up by the steroids. **He said he wouldn't be surprised if she developed diabetes down the road**. Her current sodium count is 134. She asked to have her throat sprayed with the Biotene. The doctor said he will be accepting calls from the General Hospital to discuss the case when she is transferred there. He admits this is a very difficult case.

At 1:50pm the speech therapist is checking her throat. **She advised us at this time to see the medical records department for records we will need when we are transferred to the General Hospital.** This was good advice because, with all that is going on, I wasn't thinking about paperwork just yet.

The Kidney doctor came in at 6:00pm to say the kidney function was improving. At 6:45pm they started her on Levemir, long lasting insulin. They also gave her Tylenol to control her temperature.

December 9th, at 9:00am, her sugar count is 235. Hemoglobin count is 8.2. They said it was 7.7 at the previous count. I am not sure what to make of this, except that all of her chemistry is going through a "roller coaster" period. We asked about the immunoglobulin procedure coming up. The nurse said she will check with the doctor to see when this is scheduled. At 11:15am temperature is reported as 97.7°. The rest of the vitals were good. I called for the primary doctor at 11:30am to discuss the IVIG. He will be here in about an hour. The doctors were waiting for our decision on going ahead with this therapy. Our son is in to visit today and needed some answers. He talked to the nurse leader, who then called the head nurse. The main concern is the increased weakness of his mother and the lack of action to this point. . **My son and I asked to see the head nurse. After listening to our plight the head nurse said she would arrange for us to see the Director of the hospital.**

We had a long discussion with the Director. We discussed the computer problem, doctor attitude, and nurse capability. The director was more of a public relations person. He eased us out of our tensions and assured us he would address these issues. The computer problem, he said, was rare, and he apologized for the aggravation it caused.

At 11:50am the attending nurse said she got the ok to administer immunoglobulin.

12:15pm there was a question if IVIG can be administered if there is a presence of blood in the stool. The concern over blood in the stool stems from all the medicine being administered without any solid food. By 12:35pm the primary doctor had not shown yet.

The primary doctor finally arrived at 1:30pm to discuss more options with the family. Our son was very tense, waiting for answers. The sodium count reported at this time is 151. The discussions between our son and the doctor became quite heated as the conversation did not yield any confirmed diagnosis. The feelings in the family were from the frustration of not knowing what was being treated and what the plans would be. Another consulting doctor stopped in and the situation was explained to my wife. She was able to understand the choices. The general conclusion, as suggested by clinical reports of similar cases is the administration of Immunoglobulin intravenously. We asked my wife specifically if she wanted to proceed with the current advice. She had been listening and aware of the complete conversation. She was in agreement.

At 2:50pm **the IVIG (Intravenous Immunoglobulin) was started** in the central line. I was praying again for the best. She also received some pain medication and became comfortable enough to take a nap. Despite the warnings of some possible negative reactions, by 3:50pm everything was going smoothly. At 4:10pm the nurse safely increased the dose rate according to current procedure.

By now it was well known throughout the hospital that the family was agitated. The nurse leader was also present for the increased dose rate. She noted her approval of the procedure and told us who she was assigning as a night nurse to assure us of the best of care. By 4:30pm my wife was napping again, and the nurse checked quietly to ask me if all was ok. I expressed my concern for her blood pressure at 170/72 with a heart rate of 110bpm. The nurse said she will check with the doctor in regard to different medication to help this issue. They had backed off any extra medication due to the fear of an ongoing stomach issue.

At 5:00pm my wife says the pain medicine relaxed her, but she still has some pain. The nurse just removed the Blood Pressure Machine that was malfunctioning showing an "E" on the screen. She was also waiting for a call back from the primary doctor concerning an updated decision on blood pressure medication.

At 5:30 the primary doctor, and rheumatologist, and one more doctor came into the room to discuss her situation. **They had reviewed the lab reports and confirmed muscle damage due to statins**. They still didn't offer a named diagnosis. They seemed to be cautiously guarding a full diagnosis for fear of being wrong. They had explored many names of possibilities earlier, however, because of the similarity of symptoms they didn't want to give it a "handle" yet.

Her sugar tested high at 6:00pm. The count was 244. The nurse said this was probably a result of steroids.

It was 7:40pm when she called me at home to tell me they are going to do a "scope" in the morning. I got the message on voice mail. She sounded so nasally. **Her voice was changing as her throat was swelling and the muscle was being destroyed.** We were using the Biotene regularly.

December 10, 7:30am, the day-nurse gave her a bath and washed her hair. My wife said she didn't sleep well overnight. The nurse said she was sleeping and snoring when checked. She is scheduled for an EDG (endoscopy) at 8:00am to explore the stomach and determine the reason for all the pain. She asked for more pain medication to address most of the pain in her hands, arms, and shoulders at this time. This is more likely due to the pain transmitted as the statins attack the muscle.

At 7:45am the kidney doctor increased the

intake of "free water" to help bring the sodium count down. The sodium count was 150 yesterday and is 151 today. He reported at this time that the kidney function is good. She reported her pain level to the nurse at a 6 or 7. The nurse entered it in the records and will check with the doctor. 8:40am the nurse just gave her Protonix through the IV. Protonix is a proton pump inhibitor (PPI). It can treat gastro esophageal reflux disease (GERD) and a damaged esophagus. It can also treat high levels of stomach acid caused by tumors. The nurse also gave her steroids at this time. The nurse changed the vacuum stick. This vacuum item is used to vacate the throat of mucus. This mucus build up has been an ongoing problem as my wife continues to have difficulty swallowing, and her vocal chords are getting weaker. Her nasal passage also seems to be closing because there is a distinct quality to the sound of her voice that reminds me of a person who has a cold and has been breathing helium at the same time. She sounds so vulnerable now. The nurse also took some vitals.

At 9:05am they took her for the EDG, a little

later than promised. I waited in the room down the hall from the operating room. There was coffee and Wi-Fi to keep me occupied for the next hour. At 10:30am the operating doctor told me the airway and esophagus are open and clear. There are no signs of any damage. He said there was a small red spot on the duodenum that may have caused the blood in the stool, but that seems to be on the mend. I didn't quite believe him. I got a feeling there was cause for my concern, and I would have to be on the alert as we progress. He will prescribe a new antacid to ease the area and help it to heal. As we were rolling her in her bed down the hall, I spotted my heart doctor in the hall and quickly shook his hand as we passed by. I thanked him for helping her to this point. To me he was a lifesaver.

Later, about 1:30pm, in the room, the primary doctor came in and said he prescribed a new antibiotic to control a urinary tract infection. He said her platelets are low. The sodium count is high at 154.

The nurse told us at 3:15pm a doctor was going to issue a new antibiotic for what she referred to as a UCI infection. I might have misheard her saying UTI infection. The best information I could get from her at this time is that this is a minor blood infection they can treat early. I'm kind of new at this stuff. I have to pay closer attention or ask stronger questions.

The nurse informed us they were ordering a different bed for her to help prevent bed sores. My wife is spending a lot of time on her backside now, being almost totally unable to move as the autoimmune system continues to eat away at her muscles, discharging fluid in the process.

They are hooking up the next IVIG treatment at this time. Within a few minutes the new bed showed up and they are making the switch. The methods they use are quite impressive if never seen before. The patient is always provided a slide sheet that goes between the mattress cover and the patient. This is grabbed at the corners by a team of assistants that lift and slide the patient where needed, even sideways from bed to bed.

3:20pm the infectious disease doctor came in to say he was analyzing the antibiotic needed for her application. Later the reports obtained upon discharge show approximately two pages of antibiotics tested against the blood samples for effectiveness by percentage. Resistance to antibiotics is a big concern to modern medicine.

Sugar was tested at 5:00pm and reported to be 194. They will administer quick acting insulin. Her blood pressure is 145/65, and heart rate is 101bpm. 6:10pm the nurse is bringing another smaller dose of steroids and some antacid. My wife said they gave her vitamin D3 earlier. They gave her a breathing apparatus to help her keep her lungs strong. The indicator needs to show 1500. She is getting the marker just past the 500 mark as she blows into it. Another doctor showed up to say he was ordering a series of blood tests.

Chapter Two

On December 11th I came in at 7:30am because my wife had called me at home to say she is being transported to the General Hospital. She says all her vitals were good over night. Her sugar was a little high. The blood oxygen level was perfect, but, we never had a problem in that department. 7:55am they are taking her for a CT scan of the chest, "with contrast". I am not sure what the last minute tests are going to prove other than a point of reference before leaving the Regional Hospital. **Detailed nurse to nurse telephone conversations are being conducted at this time with the new hospital as they get ready for the transport.**

At 9:15am another doctor came by to say muscle enzymes are improving. 9:30am the nurse is giving her pain medication, Diflucan (anti-fungal medication for oral thrush), vitamin D, stool softener, and Norvasc (generic: amlodipine) 10mg for high blood pressure. 10:05am, they are doing an ultra-sound on the legs. They had to cancel that because the ambulance was ready and the transport team showed at the hospital room door to take her. It seemed like a lot of last minute things they wanted for their records before she left.

This was a long ambulance ride to the downtown area, which lasted just under an hour. The ambulance was an older model. Perhaps it is just used in the transport of less than critical needs. It rattled, but worse was the smell of the exhaust fumes, very much like you would smell sitting in your car behind a city bus. With the resulting nausea we asked if there was a ventilation fan. The attendant said there was but it was noisy. We preferred it anyway and insisted the attendant turn it on.

When we arrived at the General Hospital it was about 11:30am. After a basic check-in at the Emergency Room entrance we were wheeled up to the designated room at about 12:30pm. When we got to the room the head nurse assigned to us said, **"Where have you been? We have been waiting for you since yesterday"**. With comments like that you don't know who to trust anymore. The previous hospital might have delayed the transfer to run the tests that earned them extra dollars. That is just a speculation, but we were being told at the time that they didn't get a call yet.

The regular nurses began entering information into my wife's file in the computer. Questions asked were regarding personal information and medicines we were aware of.

A team of doctors spent the first 20 minutes or so questioning our plight and treatment. The lead doctor did a strength test on her muscles. They rate the various movements on a scale of 1 to 5 by the resistance (1 being bad and 5 being the best). They sense this as they push and pull the various positions of the arms legs, and head. This is entered in her record and they can judge the progress in future testing the same way.

They weighed the patient in at 208lbs. This is an amazing contrast to someone whose normal weight was around 150lbs just a few short weeks ago. Most of this was the obvious swelling due the retention of fluids from the destruction of the muscle by the autoimmune system. That would equal almost 60 pounds of water, or nearly 8 gallons. I try to imagine trying to move my arms with a gallon jug or two tied to them, especially with most of my muscles taken away.

By this time my Brother-in-law and his wife were there to lend moral support and visit with my wife. He and I stepped out of the room where I displayed some strong emotion. He did his best to give me hope.

The doctors left the room for some initial consultation and came back a short time later with some early decisions. Based on our reports of the recent medicine and care from the Regional Hospital, they will continue the IVIG **since we think it is working**. They will further evaluate the situation as time goes on. The sodium at this time was reported at 150. That is still kind of high. This number has been an ongoing concern, and we ask for it daily since it was the first indicator that brought us to the hospital.

7:04pm the nurse came in to give her insulin. The recent sugar count is 200. The nurse also turned on the television to show us a training video on washing hands, and using the many disinfectant dispensers strategically placed throughout the hospital. They push for cleanliness to avoid the spread of infections.

The nurses then tried to install a tube feeder through the nose. It wouldn't go in right. **The swelling of the throat was pushing it back out of her mouth.** As one can imagine, this produced a gagging reaction and was extremely uncomfortable for her. They will have to talk to the doctor and take her downstairs and do it under controlled conditions. From what I am told they put a small wire in the tube to stiffen it temporarily, and watch it on an x-ray to be sure it goes in the right place.

At 7:45pm we were introduced to a "patient care tech" assigned to us for the night. At 8:00pm they installed the feeding tube in the nose. It was very stressful for her. Her heart rate went to 145. At 8:10pm they took an x-ray of the tube to be sure it was in the right place. They came in with antibiotics at 8:30pm, and decided to hold off on anxiety medication now that she has calmed down.

2:30am, the morning of December 12, the sodium count was tested at 133. That is where we want it. They administered respiratory treatment. The speech therapist was there very early in the morning of that days work. **By this time my wife was unable to swallow, and her speech is just a whisper.** At 9:30am my wife is very stressed. They changed her clothing and bedding, but all that moving around took a toll on her 208lb body. They were giving her medication through the nose feed tube and flushed it in preparation for a new pump that would administer the liquid food through the tube to the stomach. I also had to sign a consent form to let the General Hospital obtain records and information from the Regional Hospital. Of course that is necessary. 9:55am, the vitals are: blood pressure 171/61, and heart rate is 116 bpm.

11:00am, the test for blood sugar is 212. 11:20am the dietician came in to determine a preparation of a diabetes formula that will work through her feed tube. At 12:30pm the nurse brought in a new feed machine and the diabetic formula supply for the feed tube. The nurse will bring her some Tylenol for her shoulder pain. Scheduled for 4:00pm is 60mg of IV Prednisone (steroid).

1:30pm a therapist came in. He had her move her legs off the bed. He moved them gently to hang over the edge of the bed and then helped her to a sitting position. The basic reason for this treatment is to get the circulation going in a normal manner to avoid muscle atrophy and bed sores. This is a muscle affliction. What do they expect? She isn't strong enough to stand on her own this time. She showed amazing determination. They brought in a crane with a suspension saddle. They worked the saddle under her and hooked up the straps to the crane. They lifted her and wheeled over to the chair in the corner of the room, and lowered her in. The new primary doctor came in shortly after to check on her.

They moved her back to the bed with the crane

at 3:26pm. I know she was uncomfortable but, I am very proud of her courage. The saddle now stays with her. For sanitary reasons, this saddle is reused on only this patient during the patients stay.

At 4:06pm the bed pan was necessary. 4:30pm the "Charge Nurse" checked with us to answer any questions or address any issues. A few minutes later the regular nurse took the sugar count at 297. She gave her an insulin shot. Ceftriaxone (antibiotic used for mild UTI problems) was hanging on the rack empty. Vitals at 6:45pm are blood pressure 127/90 and heart rate is 119. Her temperature is 98.3°. I went home about 7:30 to clean up and restock my overnight supplies.

December 13th 8:45am I arrived. She was very uncomfortable. She needed me to adjust the bed because she felt crunched and is having trouble breathing. I got the nurses. They are paging the doctors. **She says she feels like she is suffocating**. She is very agitated and says she can't stand the bed. She asked if that other pain medicine is available, and said the Tylenol is not helping. Based on these complaints they will do a precautionary EKG and chest x-ray. 10:45am the nurse said they are bringing her a new style bed that may help make her more comfortable. A few minutes later a sugar check yielded a count of 317. The nurse returned with a shot of insulin. **Because of the unusual swelling they brought in a new wrist band and cut off the old one that was interfering with her circulation.**

She was taken for a **CT scan** around noon and returned to the room at 1:25pm. The new bed arrived, as promised, at 1:38pm and we were told they were considering different pain medication. At 2:20pm the nurse changed the protective bandages on the central line in her neck. She told us the x-ray of the feed tube shows it is in the right place. They are going to start food through the tube. A cardiologist came in at 3:00pm to tell us there was some **mild enzyme leakage from the heart** on the last test. We were told .04 was normal and hers was .07. Another neurologist doctor came in and said the CT scan was done to rule out blood clots. The scan would also show tumors, but that was negative. Small cancer cells can't be seen with this test, but she doesn't think this is going to be our problem. We can discuss this with the main neuro-muscular doctor. This test would be tied with the auto-immune testing that is being targeted at the muscle. We were informed that some of the test results they needed from the other hospital were slow in coming.

At 5:00pm the assigned nurse was setting up 60mg of IV steroids. Also insulin and Tylenol were necessary at this time. We were told an **Echocardiogram** for the heart is coming up.

At 6:30pm the primary doctor came by to discuss many of our questions. We asked about so many nagging thoughts that might have something to do with her symptoms. We asked about flu shots, heart strain with physical therapy, Gillian Barres disease, Myasitis, and auto immune problems. The doctor has made a file of this weekend with recommendations for the overseeing team of doctors when they return tomorrow. **Most of the illnesses she may have would be treated with IVIG.** The team at this hospital is the best at neuro-muscular disorders.

This doctor thinks my wife is progressing well, but added it will take a long time. The nurse wanted to give her drugs for the pain, but opted for Tylenol for now. 7:09pm the day nurse introduced the night nurse and briefed her on the medicines in front of their patient, my wife. The rotation of nurses was beginning to become apparent. They spend 12 hours on duty 3 days a week. Some run overtime while handing off shift responsibilities. They seem to prefer this schedule that allows them some free time for home, chores, etc. There also is more consistency of care with only two shifts in a 24 hour period.

December 14th, Monday, 8:30am, a skin medication person came to examine pressure points, to address possible bed sores. Her heart rate shows on the monitor at 125.

The nurse leader briefed us on the concern for my wife's shallow breaths and that is why **they put a breathing mask on her** recently. My wife filled me in. She said they came in the middle of the night and put an oxygen mask on her and scared the s*^* out of her. They told her

everything had shut down on her so they needed to give her some assistance. She thought they could have been gentler. I wasn't there at the time. I had gone home for the night. I wonder what my reaction would have been. 9:08am they are going to assess her lung function. The lungs are part of the muscle class that gets attacked by this affliction. She has to blow into a contraption to measure pressure. Her number was 1.1 last night and improved to 1.2 this morning. 9:30am she told her nurse she feels awful. The nurse is checking her eye movement, muscle movement and listening to the lungs and stomach. I'm getting the feeling **last night was quite a scare**. Maybe it was better I wasn't there.

The nurse is rolling her over to the other side to help relieve possible bed sores. She is giving her medicines, and with a test of 267 for sugar, she gave her insulin. Other medicines at this time are Protonix for her stomach. They will give her Toprol for her heart rate. During this session her heart rate dropped to 92. It was 125. She is a very sick woman.

Our daughter was visiting from out of town

today. After observing the order of things, she asked to have the Protonix set for early morning to offset the acid problems the rest of the day. They complied.

The cardiologist came by at 10.22am and says everything regarding last night's scare is looking good so far. He is not worried about a heart attack. He will be checking the echocardiogram today.

A technician came in to replace some leads on the monitor that was malfunctioning. Actually it was just a loose wire on the monitor. At 11:08 the nurse brought in a **wedge pillow to keep her on her side to avoid bed sores**. Small bed sores were beginning to show. She also put sponge boots on her feet. 11:34am blood sugar is 283; more insulin!

12:10pm a team doctor said they scheduled the diagnostic muscle test called an EMG coupled with a nerve test. This is a definitive test.

At 1:55pm the primary doctor noted the sugar count at 157. 3:15pm the cardiologist came in to tell us they will do an MRI on the heart to be sure they didn't miss anything. This concern with the heart is because this is a muscle also.

At 3:40pm the speech therapist tried some swallow therapy. My wife hasn't been able to swallow her own saliva. She needs the suction tube to relieve the accumulation of mucus deep in her throat. She constantly has to push the tube down her throat to suck the mucus out. It also helps avoid the possibility of pneumonia if these fluids build up in the lungs. The therapist wants to take an x-ray test to observe the larynx.

Another test at 4:15pm, they are doing an EKG, keeping a close watch on the heart. Sugar check at 4:50pm is 246. We know that means more insulin.

5:20pm the neurologist (head of the team) needs to find the internal bleeding that is stealing her hemoglobin. The hemoglobin and sodium has to be stabilized in order for my wife to have the proper strength to undergo a colonoscopy. They also want to do another endoscopy where they could cauterize the bleeding they suspect to find. When all of this is stabilized they can perform the EMG necessary to determine the diagnosis of her affliction once and for all. After this is all done the expected diagnosis will allow them to put an "attack plan" into place. Looking ahead they will continue steroids at lowering doses and observe the progress. The IVIG has reached its maximum dose. The rest of the plan might include Methotrexate or some similar form of **chemotherapy** later on. They refer to this as chemotherapy when it involves the immune system. My understanding of chemotherapy is coming to a hospital for some sort of chemical injection. **They use the term in a broader scope.**

December 15 a doctor and two nurses were here when I walked in this morning. They were alerted to the drop in hemoglobin again. The sodium count was high at 158. They scheduled another unit of blood to boost the hemoglobin to a safe level. Following the blood transfusion she appeared to have more color and seemed stronger. With the added strength they want to give her a barium swallow for a chest x-ray, and an MRI of the chest and maybe the hips. It seems they are manipulating the body as it struggles to correct itself.

At 11:00am a rheumatologist came by to ask many questions. He was determined to get involved and find a fix as soon as possible. He had his own notes all laid out with an almost complete byline of my wife's history before we even started to talk. I was very impressed with his determination. We completed a very thorough interview. 11:40am sugar count is 247. A couple of minutes later one of the team doctors stopped in for a routine check. At 12:30pm more blood was drawn for testing, and again at 2:00pm.

2:30pm the speech therapist says the barium swallow test she was hoping to do, is scheduled for tomorrow about 2:00pm. The blowing test my wife has been doing on a regular basis showed some improvement, going from 1.1 to 1.5. The incident **yesterday must have been a very low point**.

4:00pm the team of doctors made their regular visit. They all agree they would like to get the EMG done tomorrow since she is showing some signs of strength from the blood transfusion. No time was mentioned. The test involves electrodes placed at strategic positions at either end of the muscle. An electric shock is transmitted through the muscle to determine if it is receiving the proper message to work properly. If this occurs they can conclude that the actual weakness is in the muscle due to a necrotizing factor. The rest of the diagnosis will have to come from blood tests for certain enzymes. They also would like to schedule an endoscopy and a colonoscopy, while she is stronger, to discover and eliminate the internal bleeding problem.

4:30pm sugar count is 202 and the nurse went for the insulin. At 5:55pm the primary kidney doctor said she will increase the free water intake because the sodium count is remaining high, and this will drop the sodium. This is such a delicate balance since she is retaining water which results in the horrible swelling problem.

Later that evening, close to 7:30pm, the gastro-intestinal specialist came by to meet the patient and gather some personal information that would give him some insight as to what he will look for in the endoscopy procedure. He also explained what he is going to do. He said he would be scheduling the endoscopy after he checks out any health issues with the other doctors. He will perform the endoscopy first, then the colonoscopy if her health and strength permits it at the time. Shortly after he left she fell asleep for some well deserved rest. It seems these evenings are full of interruptions all night long. A series of nurse visits within two hour increments are always happening. They include blood draws, changing drip medicines, testing sugar levels, taking blood pressure readings and other vitals. At the "crack of dawn" someone is always there for respiratory treatments for her lungs, and they return periodically through the day. There is very little full night's sleep. It is best to catch whatever she can in-between these ordeals.

9:20pm the attending nurse is giving her 60mg of IV steroids. She will then bring insulin, if needed, when she gets the test numbers from the next check. She then went about the rest of her routine. She flushed the feed tube with water, changed the feeding bag of liquid food, and put up some new free water drip. She then listened to my wife's heart, checked foot movement and asked comfort questions. A while later a respiratory person came in to do some more "blow" exercises.   10:20pm more blood pressure and sugar level testing.

12:25am of December 16 a sonogram tests shows more than 300mg of urine being held in the bladder. Any more than that is considered unsafe and needs to be relieved. Another nurse came in to assist our nurse with the insertion of a catheter. They will give her Toprol for her heart rate. The blood sugar reading is 221, so they are giving her 4 units of insulin. They also said they will be monitoring the blood hemoglobin every 8 hours now because of the instability. 1:25am they are adding fluid to the IV line. Her blood pressure is 135/71.

The morning of December 16th at 6:00am the attending nurse is doing another bladder scan with the sonogram. My wife says she is functioning on her own for the time being. They changed the bedding. This is skillfully done by rolling the patient to one side and rolling the old bedding up to her, then putting the new bedding down on that half of the bed and forming another roll next to the old roll. Then the patient is rolled over the other way so the old roll can be completely removed from the other side, and the new portion is then rolled out flat to complete the other side. The patient then is returned to her normal position. I mention this procedure because **during this session her heart rate "red-lined", and the monitor started beeping.** With all the swelling and lack of muscle, many of these movements produced a lot of pain and trauma. After she calmed down they added a catheter because she couldn't empty her bladder naturally. Perhaps the trauma of the bed change disturbed the natural function she was experiencing earlier.

6:27am they changed the ports on the central line to prevent infection.

6:33am they are ready early to start some procedures. They will be taking her for an MRI we are told. At 6:37am the blood pressure reading is 144/65, heart rate is 99, and they tested her sugar. At 6:50am they took her away for the MRI as promised. She was back by 8:40am.

Respiratory came in at 9:10am to do another "blow" test.

A team doctor came by to tell us he got another copy of the biopsy results. He lost the first copy. He tested her strength. He performed the test at various muscle positions of the arms, hands, legs, feet and head. He assigned a "strength number" on a scale of 1 to 5 as mentioned before. She is quite tired at this time. He tells us they want to get the EMG done and compare them with the biopsy results. Her sodium is still high at 157. The hemoglobin count is slowly dropping again. This is a constant concern. They need to stop the suspected internal bleeding!

The attending nurse is drawing blood from the central line and giving her medication at 10:15am. The latest sodium count test just came back at 148. Hemoglobin is 9.9, a good number, if it will only hold. At 10:33am the nurse was giving her insulin to counter the morning count of 271.

The rheumatologist came in at 11:09am saying the muscle numbers are better. My wife should have a good response to steroids. He advised to have a lung doctor check for any problems since **they saw "cloudiness" in the upper left lung.** He examined her stomach area at this time and said he thinks a colonoscopy is scheduled.

11:20am the nurse took vitals: blood pressure 125/60, heart rate 75bpm, and temperature 96.1°. At 1:30pm sugar tested at 213. She is getting 4 units of insulin. She is told at this time she will be going for a barium swallow throat test with x-ray. 1:30pm vitals are: blood pressure 129/63 and heart rate is 88.

The team came in at 2:30pm to tell us **she is going to get that EMG now.** The head doctor will start to set it up. She was wheeled out in her bed. This was not a surprise but it seemed sudden.

The primary doctor came by, in the meanwhile, about 3:00pm and told us the CT scan of the pelvis was clear. They were not able to determine any blood leakage in this test. The test was done with and without contrast. At 3:40 the kidney doctor told us the sodium count is now 147 and they will watch it closely until it gets down to around 138-140.

She returned from the EMG at 4:00pm, only to be taken out again 30 minutes later for an MRI of the thigh.

5:15pm the internal medicine doctor came in to tell me that the muscle EMG shows the muscles were "quiet", which means the steroids have pushed back whatever inflammation there was. Healing will just take time now. 5:55pm her heart rate on the monitor is 83.

6:00pm sodium report is 150 and hemoglobin is 9.5.

December 17th, 9:45am the team of doctors arrived. They tested the various muscle movements and speech. The team leader, who performed the EMG test, repeated the message that was given to me the previous day. "The muscle response was good". They thought the muscle movement and strength in today's test was stronger than the previous day. The sodium count is 150, hemoglobin is 9.3, and the enzyme tests results are improving, meaning the muscles are healing. (I believe the "enzyme" test they refer to is what I had learned later to be the CK test).

The Physical therapy team will try to get muscle movement later today.

A throat barium test is scheduled today.

The neurology team is waiting for pathology slides to make some final determinations.

10:05am a speech therapist worked with her to try some exercises that she can try on her own later. She will make a report to the team doctors.

10:35am the physical therapy team is working with her. They brought in a machine that will help her stand. I am worried that she doesn't have the strength to endure this treatment. The machine has a large circular pipe on the top with horizontal handles extending toward the patient for the arms and grab knobs for the hands. The attendant has a control box with buttons for up and down. They proceed to sit her up in her bed and she painfully obliges. She grabs the knobs and waits for the signal. The arm section rises with the push of the button, but the speed is uncontrolled and surprises her weak shoulder muscles with so much force that **she screams in agony. I see the shoulder bones rising under her skin.** They bring it down immediately. They just don't understand this disease has eaten the muscles away and it is not done yet. Her heart rate raises so fast the red light beeps on the monitor and **the nurses rush in** from the control station. The chaos is unnerving for everyone. I am going to be forever on guard after this session. This is awful.

It is 12:03pm and the nurse is giving her insulin and blood pressure medicine. At 12:08pm the lung doctor came in to tell us there is some cloudy area in the upper left lung. This is the same news the rheumatologist gave us earlier. It is nothing to be alarmed about, he says. It just warrants watching and treating. It is probably just micro particles from trickles of saliva or mucus she has trouble vacating. This makes sense to us since she continues to need to use the vacuum suctioning tool to get the mucus out of her throat. **The muscles in her throat do not work now and she can't perform a swallow.** We need to be on guard for pneumonia.

At 2:30pm she can't seem to get comfortable.

The nurse and the aids changed some positions for her. They try wedge pillows and tilt the body for her. They also grab the "slide sheet" by the corners and bring her to the top of the bed so her waist line bends at the same place the bed does. This also rubs the top of her head on the bed because she can't hold her head up.

2:45pm the kidney doctor stopped by to say they will increase the free water to bring the sodium count down from 152. Vitals at this time are blood pressure at 131/57; heart rate is 83, with temperature at 96.5°.

3:30pm the primary doctor said she will check sodium twice a day. She ordered a scan for the possible blood leakage. She will talk to the Gastro Intestinal doctor to discuss strategy for the endoscopy.

4:00pm my wife was taken for a CT scan of the abdomen. This is the test the primary doctor ordered. They are using a contrast to be able to see any blood leakage in that area. At 6:00pm they wheeled her bed back into the room. They couldn't finish the test. They had put a cloth over her face which they do to eliminate the visual effect of the CT tunnel. The surprise was a shock to my wife and she was in such a panic they cancelled the test. She was in a confused state. Shortly after arriving back, the nurse gave her insulin. 6:10pm the blood pressure reading is 121/80,

The electric went out at 8:33pm. Some items came back on with the auxiliary power. This lasted only about a half hour. It was probably due to the storm outside.

10:00pm more vitals are checked.

At 12:36am December 18 she called for the nurse. It took a while for a response. By 12:45am someone finally showed to assist her in bathroom duties. They will scan her bladder. The attending nurse came in at 12:56am to check on her. At 1:03am the nurse returned with the bladder scanner. My wife sounded distressed. The bladder was over 500ml. They had to catheterize her. That was a full half hour after the first need to go.

After I helped with the situation the nurse then

answered some of my questions. She said the hemoglobin count at the last reading was 8.3. The sodium count was 153. They were giving my wife 5% dextrose solution, but no free water in anticipation of the upcoming endoscopy. The nurse then put moisturizer on my wife's lips. **The dryness in and around the mouth was getting pretty uncomfortable.**

At 3:13am the new hemoglobin reading is 7. They have to give her a unit of blood since 7 is the threshold. 5:03am the blood has arrived. At 5:25am the blood is started while the nurse stays with her for any adverse reaction. She is complaining of stomach pain and can't breathe. Her vitals are 100/56 blood pressure, with a heart rate of 76bpm. Sugar count is 355 at this time.

December 18th, 8:00am my wife is weak and resting. Blood pressure is 122/57. It has been a long night. 8:30am, blood pressure is 105/54, and heart rate is 76bpm. At 9:50am the medicine being given is Levemir for sugar, and Xanax to relax. They have to crush the Xanax pill and mix it with water to get it to go through the nose feeding tube. This is a constant challenge to **get the crushed product fine enough** to dissolve sufficiently to travel through this tiny 1/8" diameter tube without clogging it. When this is done, they have to follow with sufficient water to be sure that there is nothing left in the tube that will harden and compromise the passageway. Something about this seems very backward compared to the modern methods being adapted every day.

10:10am, blood pressure is 104/56, and heart rate is 73. Now that the blood transfusion has had its effect, they can concentrate on an MRI and then retry the CT scan to find the possible blood loss. The EDG (endoscopy) is scheduled for 6:45pm.

12:00pm the kidney doctor came in and checked the medicine bags on the rack regarding the attention to the sodium problem. She did not approve of the mix and straightened it out right away. Blood pressure at 12:10pm is 120/62, and heart rate is 80.

1:30pm the lung doctor came in and listened to her chest for breathing. He said to keep vacating the phlegm and mucus.

1:36pm the nurse came in to give her short acting insulin. The primary doctor came in to say **she wants the patient in ICU after the endoscopy**. Apparently they feel things aren't progressing the way they thought they should. Or maybe they fear a problem as weak as she is.

The nurse has to catheterize her to empty the bladder.

4:00pm the rheumatologist came in with his boss. The two doctors were seriously involved with questions trying to evaluate this illness as best they can.

4:40PM the nurse is doing another bladder scan to prepare my wife for her move to the ICU room where they will perform the endoscopy. The gastro intestinal doctor will perform the procedure right in the ICU room. I found this quite surprising, but later realized it was as safe as a regular operating room..

5:00pm the rheumatologist asked the nurse to draw a unit of blood for his own tests. They were also drawing blood for general counts before the endoscopy.

At 5:45pm we were just waiting for "transport" to take my wife to the ICU room and the endoscopy.

Chapter Three

OUR DARKEST HOURS

We arrived in ICU about 6:30pm, December 18.. The gastro enterologist was already there waiting for my wife. He showed me his arsenal of equipment. It was what appeared to be an enormous tool chest. It was similar to the type you see mechanics have in a very sophisticated garage where they can do almost anything to fix your car. Those tool chests are usually red in color. This one was white with many drawers and compartments and places to hang various pieces of equipment needed for the procedure. It was about the size of a small desk, only twice as high. I was told by the doctor he had a rolling program able to perform all his procedures on the spot. I can see some advantages to having your own familiar tools to do your work. I would assume fewer mistakes for one.

Before things can start she has to sign a consent form. She is unable to do this. I suggested she could get enough strength to sign an "X". We did this. Two nurses stood by to witness my wife putting her mark on the form that gave me the responsibility of making decisions.

The anesthesiologist took me aside and explained that **she was weak and they will put in a breathing tube after the procedure** to assist her breathing afterwards.   They will leave it in overnight and give her a sedative so she can sleep through the follow up time. He said anything could happen in her weak condition. I still gave the "OK". What was I supposed to do? I can see why we are in ICU, now.

When the operation was done I came to her side. She was somewhat awake and in fear of the tube they left down her throat, and coming out of her mouth. She couldn't talk but her eyes were very wide and she looked scared. She was shaking her head "No". I had to assure her this was a temporary situation to assist her while she recovers. I told her they will give her something to help her sleep, and in the morning they will remove the tube. She soon fell back into a sleep.

On December 19th at 1:30am in the morning following the endoscopy, the nurse came in and vacated the bladder through a catheter. She cleared her throat with the suction tube. She pushed the tube way down her throat. It was kind of unnerving. My wife is unable to move her arms to do this anymore. The nurse listened to her lungs. At 2:15am another attending physician checked in on her. At 6:00am there was another bladder check. They needed to keep abreast of this while she was sedated. By 7:21am she was still sleeping.

8:30am the nurse stopped the breathing assist and observed. She is doing well, breathing on her own. They will be removing the tube based on this, in about 1 to 2 hours. At 10:15am the lung doctor came in to check her. The lungs sound clear. They will take the breathing tube out. **They removed the breathing tube and watched her chest for movement. She made it!** Most of the mucus is in the throat. The gastro doctor said the stomach and the duodenum were inflamed. The ulcer in the stomach was cauterized. They will feed her with IV for now and consult when to insert another nose tube or put in a stomach feeding port called a PEG tube. She slept through most of the rest of the day.

Later as I drove home in the dark, I began to lose control of my emotions. I screamed up to the heavens, "Why don't you just take her?" Then I immediately retracted and hollered, "No, No, I don't mean it. Just help us stop this suffering."

December 20th, 10:15am, I am back. She is sleeping. The room is dark. Her hands are swollen and she sounds congested as she coughs. No one is here. 10:30am the assigned nurse came in. Blood pressure is 124/54, heart rate is 85bpm. They are adding antibiotics. The chest x-ray they took looks good. She was able to pass urine by herself at 500ml. They want to try something through the nose for the congestion. They got a lot of mucus out on the last try. The mucus situation is a constant watch. Someone has to constantly be there to clear her throat, since she has very little control of these muscles and can now barely move her own hands. She is constantly asking to have her throat sprayed with the Biotene. She also asked for lip gloss.

The pulmonary doctor is on constant watch now. I was able to oversee the computer screen and noticed the Prednisone dosage was at 60mg at 8:00 this morning.

11:08am a nurse came in to draw more blood. She is helping the nurse in charge.

At 11:45am the internal medicine doctor came in to tell me they gave her two more units of blood last night while I was gone. The hemoglobin count is now 10.2 as a result. The sodium count is 150. She is scheduled for another endoscopy and muscle biopsy tomorrow. This new blood is probably very good timing. She certainly needed all the strength she could get. All this trauma has to be taking a toll.

2:30pm, the respiratory team was here and gave her a mask to breath from for about 5 minutes. This will help keep the lungs clear and fight possible infection or pneumonia. The lab had to come in and draw blood using ultra sound to find a vein since the swelling in her arms was so swollen they couldn't locate a vein by sight. At 3:11pm they gave her an insulin shot and removed the insulin drip. She also got a diuretic to pull the water out of the system, and reduce the swelling. The nurse said she has a slight fever at 3:50pm. He turned the temperature down on the room thermostat to help her fight her fever.

December 21, 8:10am, one of the team doctors reported the platelet count at 84 (normal range is 150-350), sodium was 142, and hemoglobin was at 8.2. Blood pressure is 158/60, and heart rate is 103bpm. She looked pretty good at this time. They took her out of the room for a muscle biopsy. I went with her and stood by the bed in the hallway, waiting for an operating room to be ready. The doctor came out and explained a simple procedure. They will make a small incision in her upper arm and remove a strand of the muscle. They will cut with the grain of the muscle to avoid large scars and promote easier healing. Then they will suture the cut and it will be over.

The room was ready in a few minutes. The procedure didn't take long.

  We are back in the room at 10:15am. The nurse said they are trying to eliminate a possible diagnosis of Myasthenia Gravis disease (a disease which affects the thyroid and the lung). She is reporting hemoglobin holding at 9.1 on the last two readings. Platelets are 84. She will ask for a complete blood count to get a safe reading before another endoscopy scheduled for 2:00pm. 11:29am, the blood pressure is 144/74, and the heart rate is 80bpm. 11:30am the nurse set her up with the bedpan. They are giving her potassium, and will be drawing blood. Sugar is 246. Temperature is 97.8°. Bladder scan is 400ml.

  12:30pm the lung doctor examined her and said everything sounded good. He wants her to do breathing exercises with a sucking machine to expand her ability to inhale. 1:50pm she underwent a breathing session with the respiratory technician to open the lungs and provide medicine to prevent the onset of pneumonia. He brought in a sucking machine. It is actually just a plastic tube shaped tower, about

6 or 7 inches tall with a mouthpiece. It is calibrated to indicate the level of sucking power the patient can generate at any one time as the inside cylinder moves under her pressure. They will leave it with her to use whenever she wants to keep her lung strength. She needs to do this often.

1:55pm the kidney doctor says her sodium count is 151. They ordered potassium to boost a low potassium reading. At 2:07 the nurse said the platelet count went lower and hemoglobin is 9.2. We are happy the hemoglobin seems to be holding.

2:50pm the primary doctor of internal medicine says they will keep her stable for the next couple of days while they await the biopsy results. So we will just bide our time, for awhile.

3:26pm the nurse took her temperature at 98.2°. They are adding platelets to prepare for her upcoming endoscopy and PEG tube (Percutaneous endoscopic gastrostomy tube). It is an endoscopic medical procedure in which a tube (PEG tube) is passed into a patient's stomach through the abdominal wall, to provide a way of feeding when oral intake is not practical.

3:58pm the nurse gave her steroids, and something for blood pressure. 4:02pm temperature is 98.1°. 4.24pm temperature is taken again at 98.2. Her temperature and blood oxygen level always seems to be good, but they watch it closely.

6:30pm I left to have dinner in the hospital cafeteria, as they took her for the endoscopy and PEG tube placement. I returned as soon as I could and waited in the waiting room for the procedure to finish. I watched a couple young children push chairs together so they could play. They were there with their mother waiting for word of a loved one.

At 9:05pm I called back to the room to get an update on the endoscopy. It had been quite awhile. They said they had delayed the procedure while waiting for platelets from the pharmacy. The procedure was successful. They said the ulcer stopped bleeding and showed signs of healing. They put the PEG tube in.

12:01am **she is calling "help me"**. She had

some trouble breathing. The nurses came in to help calm her down. What a scary feeling. She was probably coming down from the anesthesia and trauma of the PEG tube procedure.

December 22, 4:45am I woke. **She is calling out**. The nurse button was off the bed. She was uncovered and no one was around. I found the button unit for her. This was so important to her since she was helpless without it, unable to move, and very weak speech. The nurse in charge said she was called away to help another nurse. I told her to be sure the nurse button is by her hand at all times since she is too weak to yell out. The nurse gave her pain medication at this time. I am glad I was there at that moment.

4:55am the lights came on. The heart rate had dropped to such a low level that set off an alarm. The nurses came in quickly. They woke her up and kept calling to her to get the heart rate going again. I told the nurse leader to keep a closer watch on her at this delicate time. The nurse suctioned her throat with a smaller tube. It cleared her better but there was some pinkish

bloody look to it. **I was getting very worried**.
After the nurse left I consoled my wife. **She said "I
don't think I can't go on"**. I told her we have
turned the corner, **"you can make it"**. This was
looking pretty bad.

5:15am she is calmer now. I am thinking the
anesthetic took a toll on her weakened condition
last night.

7:15am the nurses are attending to her. She
was quite uncomfortable. They did their check-
ups and tests. **She seems very weak**. 7:45am a
technician administered a respiratory treatment.
He listened to her lungs and had her take a deep
breath and cough. He used a mask this time to
administer the breathing and lung medication.
Afterwards she asked for the Biotene spray.

8:10am the doctor in charge of critical care
came in to evaluate her present condition. The
day nurse will give her water. The gastro
intestinal doctor prescribed Pedialyte after the
endoscopy. This sends the sodium up. The water
will bring the sodium down from the current
count of 153. What a conflict. Hemoglobin was
8.1 and now is 8.9. The nurse wants to get her

into her chair later this morning. 8:22am she is having a much needed sleep.

9:11am the pulmonary doctor checked on her. He is concerned about the sodium level remaining so high. The free water will help. He will come back in an hour to observe the progress. 9:20am, the nurse is taping the belly to protect the PEG tube. She is going to have the lift team put her in the chair.

10:00am the internal medicine doctor came by to say the "numbers are stable". Sodium is a little high at 153. He talked to our son from the room on Skype. He told him the recent swelling could be symptomatic of recent trauma from the last procedure. He deferred the discussion of muscle problems to the neurology group. That team should be showing up here soon. As much as our son pressed for answers, there isn't much this doctor can add concerning the specialty questions.

The nurse mentioned Myasthenia Gravis disease which is a chronic autoimmune neuromuscular disease that has varying degrees of weakness of the skeletal (voluntary) muscles of the body. My thoughts are the EMG would suggest otherwise. However, it is good to pay attention to suggestions. Each nurse has a thought to offer.

Earlier in the morning the attending nurse had ordered a special bed for my wife. It arrived a little after 10:00am and they switched the patient to the new bed. At 10:40am the nurse proudly turned on this new bed. The idea is the extreme shaking designed into this bed is supposed to help bring up fluid from the lung. It shook for 10 minutes. I asked my wife if she was aggravated by this and she said it was all right. It was hard to watch. She looked very uncomfortable as it visibly vibrated her whole body.

12:00pm the lung doctor said they are concerned about muscle weakness as it may apply to breathing down the road. I wasn't surprised at this, given the many visits she gets from the respiratory team. The sodium and sugar they can control. The muscle function is another matter. It sounded logical to me. I feared this possibility.

12:10pm the discharge supervisor came by to talk about long term care. This is a scary thought.

Are they assuming she won't get any better? I listened, but felt this was a little premature. She isn't going anywhere for a while from my point of view. Why do they do this to us?

1:10pm the nurse changed the patient's boots. These sponge boots are to keep the feet elevated off the bed and prevent sores. Hemoglobin is reported holding at 8.8.

1:45pm the rheumatologist came in. He was discussing the case with his superior and is waiting for all the tests he ordered to come in. They are checking Lyme disease also, per my request. He ordered 2 more blood samples at this time.

1:50pm physical therapy came in to see how she sits and balances. They were quite rough with her. They sat her up but I felt they were careless with the newly placed PEG tube in the way. It would be better if it were wrapped to her stomach in some way. They insisted they do this all the time after an operation. It is best to get the circulation going right away. My fear is they are not familiar with this rare affliction. The muscle tissue isn't there, as it is in most other cases. The tissue is like *jello*. This is a rare case and they are treating it with routine procedures. I don't agree with them.

2:20pm the rheumatologist came back to tell us that Lyme disease is ruled out.

3:15pm, the rheumatologist came in again. Some of the blood tests are back. He said ferritin is high. It is a protein found inside cells that stores iron so your body can use it later. A ferritin test indirectly measures the amount of iron in your blood. She has a low ESR rate. The erythrocyte sedimentation rate (ESR), also called a sedimentation rate or Westergren ESR, is the rate at which red blood cells sediment in a period of one hour. It is a common hematology test, and is a measure of inflammation. He thinks HLH is a possible blood disorder. When I looked this up, I felt there were not enough criteria to confirm this idea. **The pathologist biopsy showed necrotizing large tissue death** which he is thinking could be induced by HMG statins.

The nurse sent for thyroid tests and some others.

December 23 8:00am **the hematologist is reporting anemia**. The hemoglobin and platelets are low. **They are considering a bone marrow biopsy**. The muscle biopsy showed clotting in the muscles, called infarction. Hemoglobin is 9(it should be 12 and above they are telling me). The team doctors will come back to discuss the need for the bone marrow biopsy and what to expect.

9:35am the pulmonary doctor just came in. **My wife's cultures show E Coli and pneumonia symptoms.** They are trying choose an antibiotic that will take care of both. If the E Coli is just in the urine, the antibiotic should take care of it. They are still hoping to do a colonoscopy to rule out other possibilities.

10:04am the nurse set up an albumin drip to help pull some water from her body. Her hands are so swollen.

The infectious disease doctor says that Meropenem (antibiotic) is in short supply so they will use Tobramycin for the UTI. Cefepime antibiotic will be used to fight the lung infection which is **not pneumonia so far**. They will do the bone marrow biopsy tomorrow. He said one of his partners will be by later to check on her.

The internal medicine doctor came by to say many doctors are in on this case. They have a group meeting everyday to determine the next strategy. She is a priority case.

11:40am the nurse says they want a CT scan of her abdomen. Cefepime antibiotic is scheduled for 12:00noon and another dose at 11:00pm. She brought in the Cefepime at 11:25am to hook it up to the IV. At 2:16pm she reported that the TSH (thyroid stimulator hormone) was low at ".01". This is a new statistic to us.

The leading doctor of the team came in at 3:05pm to say they are looking at a diagnosis of **Necrotizing Myopathy**. I had to look that one up and do my research.

3:15pm the physical therapy team came in and sat her up. She tried very hard to cooperate but was so very weak.

Three doctors came by today with various reports. **The pathology report confirms muscle damage by statins**. The blood is not balancing so they want to do more checking when the bone marrow biopsy is finished. She is mildly sedated. She asked to have her throat sprayed with the moisturizer. This is an ongoing request.

The infectious disease doctor came in and repeated the information of a bone marrow biopsy scheduled for tomorrow. He says he doesn't think her affliction is HLH, but they want to see why she is anemic. He mentioned the use of **smaller vials for blood draw** might be better. He said it's possible her marrow isn't reproducing the blood fast enough to withstand all the draws in the larger vials.

8:11pm the night nurse is giving her pain medication now. Then she will give her contrast through the PEG tube so she is ready for the CT scan of her abdomen. At 8:40pm an assistant came in to give her a bladder scan: It is 400+, they catheterized her, and she is ready to go off to the CT scan. 9:50pm she is just back from the CT scan and very sleepy.

11:50pm she woke up from a dream. She was calling to me. She told me she wanted all the street lights off. She was very insistent and appeared to be awake. I hugged her face and calmed her down. She focused on me and said she realized she must have been dreaming. Then she said, "I'm sorry". It was such a helpless situation.

December 24, Christmas eve, 4:10am the nurse gave her medication and vacated her throat. 6:00am a doctor came in to talk to the nurse. Sugar tested at 198, and the last sodium count was 145. Blood cultures are positive for infection. They want to test vein blood to determine the source.

6:30pm the doctor on duty took her off dextrose and increased the free water.

7:48am a neurology doctor gave her a general examination. He said the bone marrow biopsy will determine which medicine they are going to use to heal her condition. The information keeps coming.

8:00am a tech could not find a vein to draw blood for the test. He said they will have to do it by sonogram. 8:20am the nurse is flushing the central line and then will draw blood for other tests. She is going to administer the antibiotics Tobramycin and Cefepime now. Pain medication is not due until 8:50am. She continues to complain of stomach pain. Sugar at this time is 165. Platelets dropped from 130 to 23. The nurse gave her pain medication at 9:20am.

9:21am the neurologist, head of the team of doctors, examined her. She reported they are anxious to see the results of the bone marrow biopsy. White cell count is low and platelets are low.

9:50am someone came in to do a sonogram to draw vein blood. 10:00am the nurse told us the bone marrow biopsy is scheduled for 1:00pm. 10:15am the nurse is giving her Tobramycin. White blood count is reported at 4.2(normal is 4.4), platelets are 33(normal ,they tell me, is 140+). The comparisons were provided by the nurse. She told us the name of the pathologists who will do the bone marrow biopsy. 12:30pm the nurse is catching up on the medicines and will put in a Foley catheter (12mm) which is more permanent. The stress of constant catheterization is causing irritation and inflammation. (I wonder if they even thought that they have been doing this to her for a month now.) Sugar tested at 193.

It is just past 1:00pm and we are waiting in the hallway for the biopsy. The biopsy was explained by the prevailing doctor. My wife told me, "Just as long as they knock me out". I told the doctor what she said. He assured her the area will be numbed and she will be sedated. The procedure was relatively simple and quick. They drilled a small hole in her hip. By 2:30pm everything was done and she was back in her room.

5:55pm I was told they were going to give her a strong antibiotic called Primaxin. I researched this on the internet and found the description to indicate ingredients called imipenem/cilastatin. I immediately drew fear when I saw the statin indication. Once I got through to the infectious disease doctor he reassured me that the cilistatin is not the statin related to the chemical combination found in cholesterol medicine. At 6:00pm the nurse administered the Primaxin and pain medication.

December 25th, 10:30am, it's Christmas morning. The nurse gave her Tobramycin and Primaxin. The hemoglobin count is 9.2, platelets are 32. The nurse asked the pulmonary doctors to discuss options for the central line currently in the patient's neck. At 1:14pm the infectious disease doctor examined my wife.

Our daughter brought in some mistletoe. She used my camera to take a picture of me giving my wife a Christmas kiss under the mistletoe. The nurse gave my wife Primaxin at 2:42pm.

4:24pm the internal medicine doctor came in to discuss options for something other than the central line in her neck. He would like to make a serious try to get something started in her arm. I told my wife I was trying to get that uncomfortable thing removed from her neck as a Christmas present to her. Ultra sound was ordered for the arm. At 5:00pm the ultra sound technician showed up to study her arm for the possibility of some entry there. He was not very successful.

At 7:00pm the nurse gave her Fentanyl. This is drug used to help prevent pain after surgery or other medical procedure. It is a potent, synthetic opioid. At 7:30pm the nurse gave her a suppository. At 9:45pm the nurse gave her stool softener to encourage some bowel movement. She also gave her antacid and long acting and fast acting insulin.

Another internal medicine doctor came in at 10:00pm to continue the discussion of the central line choices. The nurse and some helpers cleaned her up for the night.

December 26th. 5:40am. the procedure of changing bedding and giving medication lasted until 6:12am. More medication was given to her at 7:45pm.

The leading team doctor came in at 9:50am. We were told at this time there is no lab report on the bone marrow yet. The doctor also told us of some choices of autoimmune therapy. **Methotrexate and cyclosporine are considerations**. This would be done together with the IVIG (immunoglobulin) treatments. This is, of course, if all the tests support their suspected diagnosis of Necrotizing Myopathy.

The nurse gave my wife longer lasting pain medication at 10:05am. The primary doctor came in a few minutes later to discuss changing the central line. They can make an access near the collar bone (some call it a tunnel line) that can remain for a long period of time. Our nurse had made the same suggestion earlier. The doctor wasn't aware of the future need for IV treatments, but considered this to be the determining factor. The new line also makes sense for future access. He will talk to the leading team doctor to confirm the future IV needs. After he left, the nurse returned for a general check of the patient. At 11:00am the primary doctor returned to say the tunnel line (or Medi-port) is possible. They seem to throw these terms around. I am never sure which one I am dealing with. For sake of discussion, when I try to talk to the doctors I am referring to different names. They know what I mean, but don't correct me.

The nurse gave her more insulin at 11:55am. She reported hemoglobin count at 7.8, sodium at 140, and platelets 45.

The nurse from the gastro enterologist team came in at 1:00pm to examine her PEG tube.

2:30pm the rheumatologist told us they have to clear her of any infections before any previously discussed treatments can be done.

December 27th 9:45am the nurse from one of the team doctors said the culture they were waiting for yesterday is negative. Now they need the bone marrow report. It seems so long when waiting for reports. The time goes by so slowly anticipating these things.

10:00am platelet count is 56, sodium 142, hemoglobin 8.2, and sugar 227. Today she has counts approaching normal, she seems more comfortable. Her blood counts are better all the way around. She does not need a lot of pain medicine. Her breathing is fuller. I feel like it is a better day. She needs her Biotene spray and lip gloss.

11:35am the nurse tells me they have discontinued one of the antibiotics, Tobramycin. Now they are just giving her Primaxin (more good news?). At 11:50am the infectious disease doctor came in to confirm they are down to one antibiotic. Blood tests are showing all is under control. Good news!

12:45pm a doctor came in to explain the port they want to put in her vein.

At 2:40pm the nurse gave her long lasting pain medicine (Norco-a combination of acetaminophen and hydrocodone), and at 3:50pm gave her blood pressure medicine called Toprol. At 8:00pm she was given Ativan (for anxiety).

The next morning December 28th at 7:15am the nurse gave her morphine for pain. Her stomach is still bothering her. I asked for a binder on the PEG tube. It has been the source of pain in the past. Before giving the pain medicine they routinely ask for a pain level from the patient on a scale of 1 to 10. About an hour later she gave the patient prevacid, and Solu-Medrol (an anti-inflammatory glucocorticoid, which contains methylprednisolone steroid).

10:15am the nurse gave more medication. My

wife got Xanax, Toprol, and Norco. Numbers at this time are: hemoglobin 8.1, sugar 165, sodium 143, and platelets 71. A doctor came in at 11:20am to say infections are clear.

12:28pm the nurse checked her temperature at 98.3°, checked her for pain, and tested sugar at 163. She will prop her up from the side in a half hour. At 2:40pm a team doctor came in to say another session of Immunoglobulin can start next Monday. Immunosuppressant will start as soon as the bone marrow answers are addressed.

5:00pm, the nurse gave her Toprol, antibiotics, morphine, and steroids. The infectious disease doctor came in to say the bone marrow biopsy shows no cancer. We need to get through the antibiotic that was started. We have 7 days left. We then can start immunosuppressant therapy with the IVIG (intravenous Immunoglobulin).

7:30pm the night nurse is checking the last dose of Xanax. She is giving her Norco pain medicine. She determined it is too soon for more Xanax. The next dose is not due until 10:00pm.

December 29th, 10:00am the nurse is reporting sodium at 140, hemoglobin 8.0 (this seems to be slipping again), platelets are 92, and sugar a respectable 116. At 12:38pm the nurse is giving her Robitussin, Primaxin, and Norco.

The rheumatologist came in at 2:30pm to discuss some conclusions. **They are definite on "Necrotizing Myopathy"** and have 3 possible causes. **The most suspected is statins.** He said to look up Rituximab as a possible immunosuppressant we can use. One of the side effects is brain damage. I was feeling very reluctant to use something like that no matter how rare the risk. After all, she still has her wits, and mind. We don't want to gamble on losing that, too. *This affliction is also supposed to be rare.*

4:10pm physical therapy came in to get her into the chair. This is done by rolling her around on the bed until they can position the sling under her. The "crane" lifts her in the sling and puts her down in the chair with the sling in place. By 5:10pm she requested to go back to the bed. The duration is very tiring. Her sugar checked out at

131 at this time.

6:00pm the primary doctor said he will watch the hemoglobin closely for us. 6:08pm the nurse gave her Norco, morphine, and Robitussin.

December 30th, 6:30am the nurse gave her morphine and reported hemoglobin count at 8.3. She mentioned that Carafate can be given for acid stomach. Our daughter came to visit and took over for me at 10:00am while I took a break at home. 1:45pm was a respiratory treatment. 2:13pm she received more morphine and Norco. 4:00pm therapy came in to work on the ankles, knees, and legs. 4:50pm, platelets are 102 (up and down like a roller coaster), sugar 172, hemoglobin 8.3, temperature 98.3°, and sodium 136. It seems that things are starting to stabilize. The nurse gave her Xanax, Toprol, and a suppository.

December 31, New Year's Eve, 8:20am, the nurse took temperature at 99.2°, and sugar is 153. She gave her steroids, and carafate, and a low dose of insulin. She asks for some Biotene spray for her dry mouth.

At 8:55am two doctors came in to see my wife. I asked them to watch the hemoglobin closely. They will also watch the respiratory situation. They prefer to **move her out of ICU** at this time to avoid any bad infections that sometimes are prevalent in these settings. I feel comforted knowing that they think she is ready for this move. Respiratory team came in at 9:00am for her treatment. 1:45pm sugar reading is 130. The nurse gave her Robitussin and Primaxin. 2:00pm the primary doctor said the IVIG can start Monday. They will start the immunosuppressant medicine after the IVIG and the biopsy results are complete.

2:45pm a throat specialist came in to practice swallow exercises. She gave her a series of exercises that can be done on her own. There were about 3 pages printed on regular 8" X 11" stationary. They practiced 12 swallows.

Chapter Four

WE ARE OUT OF I.C.U.

It's New Years Eve and we arrive at a new semi-private room. We graduated from ICU. At 4:30Pm the assigned nurse came in to orient herself with the new patient. After working up her records on the computer station, she takes my wife's temperature at 98.0°, and blood sugar tested at 131. The primary doctor for this station came by at 6:00pm to say the platelets are coming back. The bone marrow test was good. The possibility of HLH is ruled out. The nurse came back to give my wife Robitussin at 6:47pm. I told her I would like to stay the night in the chair. The chair was squeezed between the bed and the back wall. I could barely get my hands around to the handle to raise my feet. I explained to the nurse that my wife needed constant suctioning to clear the phlegm from her throat, since she has no swallowing muscles. Plus I was constantly spraying Biotene in her mouth to relieve the dryness. She produced no syliva.

The crowded conditions were evident. There was a "tree" of metal hooks to hold all the medicine and fluid bags required. This 'tree' was pushing out the curtain that divided the semi private area. There was a monitor machine also in the way of the "tree". The suctioning controls were on the wall behind all of this. There were bags and boxes of pads, sponges, booties, apparatus forwarded from ICU, and various other items including the breathing aids, all piled up on the window shelf. The room was crowded and confusing. This is not the best environment for someone as sick as my wife.

After the 7:00pm nurse shift change, we waited to meet our night nurse. She came in about 7:45pm to meet us. She was a very experienced middle aged woman who was quite interested in giving us the best care advantage. She looked over our crowded area and expressed her thoughts saying, "this won't do". She left the room and returned about a half hour later with some surprising news. She told us she located a private room just down the hall and has someone cleaning and disinfecting it now. It would be a little while before we could move, but she encouraged us to be patient.

About 9:30pm we were moved into a private room. The room appeared to be recently renovated with new equipment outlets, new flat screen TV, and looked sparkling clean. There was a 7 foot couch at the end of the room for me to sleep on. The nurse that arranged the switch could not remain our nurse since the area had its own assigned crew. There was plenty of room for all of the equipment she needed to improve her situation. The room would prove to be better suited to the attendees who had to constantly gather around her.

Sugar was checked at 10:00pm. The count is 230. The night nurse gave her insulin, blood pressure medication, and heart rate medication. Later that night we watched the flash of New Year's Eve fireworks out the window. I relayed the visuals I could see down the side near the bridge over the water. It was a somber night given the fact she could no longer scratch her own nose. **The muscles in her body had all been**

consumed, and she lay there with trust in my support, and faith in the future. The future was so uncertain.

On January 1, 2016, Friday, 8:00am the neurology doctor came in to tell us they will start another IVIG infusion on Monday. They want a doctor to examine her lungs after learning that she coughed all night. She can't seem to get the phlegm out. The suction machine was the only way. It was very hard for either one of us to get a decent night's sleep with all the attention she needs. This private room is absolutely necessary.

A little later the nurse reported blood in the stool. She will hold back on stool softener. At 10:30am a doctor came in and using a stethoscope heard some "rattling" in the upper chest. No more than 5 minutes later they came to take an x-ray of her chest. This is done conveniently in the room while she stays in the bed. Thank goodness for the big room. The x-ray equipment is quite bulky. The plate is put behind her, the machine in the front. The tech stands to the side and pushes the button to take the picture. I stand outside the room for a few seconds when he pushes the button, and then he calls me in.

At 11:15am she received antibiotics and Robitussin. They call it Robitussin for our convenience because we might not be aware of the generic name Guaifenesin. It helps to loosen phlegm. Sugar tested at 196, Hemoglobin is 8.5, and sodium is holding at 133. Just before noon the internal medicine doctor came in to reassure us they will start the IVIG on Monday. He is going to make sure all infections are clear.

Therapy team moved her to her chair at 1:00pm. She was absolutely unable to help them as they prepared her harness and then crane lifted her to the chair. She is so determined to get better she endured the chair until 4:30pm. After returning to bed she received her metoprolol for her heart. The nurse changed some of the tubing for feeding and tested her sugar at 186. Just before 6:00pm the blood pressure was checked at 141/85, and 90bpm, and carafate and Robitussin were given.. Our daughter was in for a visit and I accepted the time she gave me to go home and freshen up for tomorrow.

January 2, at 5:30am she was given more carafate, robitussin, insulin and steroids. At 8:00am she received Primaxim, Metoprolol, a little mouth spray, and morphine. Her blood pressure was 135/51. With the help of her medicines the blood pressure has been quite stable. Because the heart is a muscle, it is important to keep things in check. We started propping her elbows up with a pillow under each. This way she was able to hinge her arm toward her face to scratch or wipe her own nose. This was a small step in the right direction, but it wasn't easy for her. Around noon she got more Robitussin. She also got one of her regular breathing treatments. Later that night her blood pressure was 114/46 which I thought was kind of low. I was reassured that it was good. Her sugar was good at 136. More medicines were given at midnight. It seems there isn't any way to get a full night's sleep.

January 3rd at 6:30am she gets more Robitussin. Sugar is 143, temperature 98.3°, and blood pressure 124/46. However, the hemoglobin has been slipping. They are still in fear of blood loss somewhere in the digestive tract. There will have to be another endoscopy to check that old ulcer. The feeding system leaves the stomach vulnerable to the harshness of the medicines. There isn't sufficient bulk and fiber that natural food provides. The gastro doctor checked on her and ordered a unit of blood for a transfusion to bring the hemoglobin count up. We are constantly fighting the hemoglobin levels which are essential to stabilizing her. He did not like seeing a pus area around the incision. At 11:00am her sugar was 118(good), platelets count at 89(low), sodium is 133(just right), White cell count 4.6, and hemoglobin was 6.7(very low). The threshold for transfusion is 7. Anything lower is considered dangerous. However, it is interesting that her blood oxygen count was always 98% or above.

At 12:30pm she was transported to another floor for a CT scan of her GI tract. This was done by moving her in her own bed, since too much changing would take even more energy that she didn't have. She gets very weak when the hemoglobin count is so low. After she got back they took her vitals again (138/57bp, platelets 77 and 98.3° temperature). The blood arrived at the same time and they hooked it up and transfused her through the tunnel line (med port). A nurse must stay with her at least 15minutes during the beginning to see if the patient has any adverse reaction to the foreign blood. They take a blood sample earlier in the day and match the properties with the donor as best they can to minimize any chance of an adverse reaction.

The procedure of watching in the beginning is a precaution. While the blood was entering her veins she was given a lung treatment by a respiratory technician about 4:00 o'clock. After he left they tested her sugar to be 113.

4:55pm and the blood is done. They removed the empty bag and gave her steroids, carafate, and Robitussin. At 5:55pm we are told the gastro doctor has scheduled another endoscopy for 4pm Monday. Another vitals check shows blood pressure 136/51 and temperature 98.1°. Later that night, just before 10:00pm, the nurse gave her Miralax, and Gatorade for electrolytes in preparation for the endoscopy in the morning. About midnight she woke up in pain. The Charge nurse came in to help my wife's night nurse. They concluded she is constipated. They had the medical answers ready and with the consult of a doctor's permission they went to work to relieve her symptoms. They gave her a stool softener, Xanax to calm her down, more morphine, and a suppository. They sent her immediately for and x-ray and a CT scan which showed a build up.

Monday morning, January 4th, the new nurse is on duty. It is 9:00am and my wife wants to know the options for bowel relief. Her sugar count is 110, a good start for the day. Potassium is low at 3.3 (normal is 3.5-5.0) so they will give her a potassium pill which will have to be crushed and dissolved in water to get it in the PEG tube without plugging it up. More morphine is due. My wife agreed to an enema. Her hemoglobin is reported at 8.1 which will permit the endoscopy to occur. They gave her carafate first and waited 20 minutes before giving her Metoprolol and stool softener. The carafate coats the stomach lining before introducing other harsh medicines. At 10:00am the nurse turned off the Gatorade. She gave her Metoprolol and potassium. She said they will not give her the stool softener at this time since the color is red and might interfere with the conclusions of the upcoming endoscopy.

10:35am and Physical Therapy team is here to sit her up on the bed. They had her sit for 5 minutes. She was very weak, but cooperated because of her drive to get better. The team neurologist came in at 11:00am to acknowledge the IVIG starts today. She says there is no problem finishing the Primaxim even though any infections are clear. They will test for the presence of JC virus to weigh the risk of using Rituximab for chemotherapy down the road. The JC virus could interfere with the Rituximab and cause brain damage. (Progressive multifocal leukoencephalopathy [PML] is the rare and often fatal disease characterized by damage to the white matter of the brain. It is caused by the John Cunningham *virus* [JCV], a common *virus* usually kept under control by the immune system.) One of the side effects of Rituximab is brain damage.

Although rare, every precaution is taken. I was very nervous about considering this drug, since my wife's wits were still intact and I didn't want to risk further heartache. I was told the side effects are very rare. I responded: "So is the affliction she has from the statins!" I was not willing to take the chance and I had long discussions with my wife as to what drug we might want to settle on. We had to choose from about 6 suggested drugs to keep the immune system under control while she healed and grew muscle back. The combination of one of these drugs with the steroids and the IVIG was the current treatment as described in many journals. Of course the doctors have little experience with this affliction and meet on a daily basis to discuss my wife's very difficult case.

The transport team showed up before 2 o'clock to take her to the operating room for her endoscopy. 2:30pm she was wheeled into the recovery room in her bed to wait for the operation. The nurse there tested her sugar at 44. He was very concerned and immediately administered glucose to bring it up to safe level. She was transported to the operating room at 3:30pm for the endoscopy. I was informed by the anesthesiologist that they will watch her very closely, but she is very weak, and things can go wrong. I waited in the recovery room for her return. **At 4:15pm I was told they took the PEG tube out. It was infected.** Her temperature was 97.7°. Upon her return to the recovery room at 4:48pm the sugar tested at 51, which was still too low, so they gave her dextrose through the IV port.

5:30pm and we are back in her room. The nurse asked us to leave while they inserted a nose feed tube. I expressed my concern. I told them the last time someone tried it didn't work because of the swelling in her throat. The nurse assured me she has done this many times and knows what she is doing. I've heard that before! A while later they came out to tell me it didn't go as expected. I wasn't surprised, but also angry. They will have a doctor do it under a fluoroscope to be sure it enters the throat passage correctly. I am beginning to believe I am the only one who can fight on her behalf. She is too weak to fight. The nurses and staff go by the manual. This is their job. This is my loved one. I will be putting my foot down in the future.

The nurse said the PEG tube reportedly was rubbing on the GI wall and created another ulcer. The doctor cauterized the ulcer during the endoscopy and they will have to wait while it heals before deciding to put another PEG tube in. **This is a step backwards.**

The night nurse and a tech tested her sugar at 70. Blood pressure at 128/52. This was done about 9:15pm. At 9:30pm the nurse gave her some Benadryl to calm her for the IVIG to follow. This is standard procedure. At 9:45 the nurse came back to prepare for the IVIG. At 9:56pm the IVIG was ready and she started the first drip. She said she had to leave the room and asked me to watch for 15 minutes. She didn't tell me what to watch for nor what to do if something happened. She had to attend to another patient. The protocol for the IVIG calls for a trained nurse to be there for the first 15 minutes. I like this nurse but I wasn't pleased with this move. The nurse returned in 17 long minutes to increase the flow. All went well, but not without anticipation.

January 5 the morning vitals are: Potassium

3.2(they were now worried about these levels), sodium 129, hemoglobin 8.1, sugar 70(low), platelets 70, and white cells 3.2. At 8:50am, the gastro doctor was on the nurse's phone as she handed it to me. He apologized for his busy schedule, and filled me in on his findings. He told me he had to remove the PEG tube, but found no abscess. However there was infection. He cauterized the area where the ulcer may have bled. The nurse will swab the PEG wound and send it to the lab for cultures. They will stay on top of it until she is ready for a new PEG tube.

The primary doctor stopped in at 9:30am and we reviewed the latest information on the peg tube. He was hoping they would have swabbed internally while they were in there to determine the extent of the infection. He said he wants speech therapy to get involved to get the swallowing and voice going. She can only speak in a whisper at this time, and of course, cannot swallow. We can only keep her mouth moist with the Biotene.

I asked to see the Head nurse at this time. My anger and frustration had been brewing for quite a while, and I thought it was about time I opened my mouth and told somebody what was on my mind. At 9:45am the Head Nurse came into the room to see me. I told her of the rough treatment my wife received in ICU by the physical therapy team. I told her that on December 22, I believed they tore the skin by the PEG tube which led eventually to the infection. I demonstrated that she has no muscle. I held my hands in front of me with the fingers pointing toward each other and intermixed. I said this is our muscle. Then I took one hand away, leaving the other hand up with the fingers spaced. I said this is her muscles, there isn't much left to hold together. We have to treat her more delicately while she heals. I also told her about some of the decisions that came down from ICU, such as smaller blood tubes so as not to drain her blood supply, making her weak. It was thought, due to the results of the bone marrow study, that she is not producing more blood fast enough. She also is supposed to get smaller catheters. I asked why this information doesn't follow on the computer with the patient. It's like putting the wrong size shoes on someone. The head nurse was supportive and assured me she would pass on this information. In fact she said it gave her fortification for a point she has been pushing with the software team regarding their computer program. She would like to see a type of "front page" on the patient's information.

11:25am the sugar count is 147. At 2:30pm they gave my wife potassium. Temperature at 2:40pm is 98.0°, blood pressure 141/55. An enema is given at 3:30pm. 4:00pm the sugar reading is 140.

The infectious disease doctor came in at 4:50pm and said he will check the culture on the infection at the PEG tube site, and decide what antibiotic to use. The antibiotics develop resistance to various infections in the body. The Lab test can be 2 pages long showing the results of cultures run against 20-30 different antibiotics and the percentage of effectiveness before deciding which one will do the job.

At 5:30 they gave her an IV steroid like Prednisone, called Solu Medrol. Solu-Medrol is an anti-inflammatory glucocorticoid, which contains methylprednisolone sodium succinate as the active ingredient. Glucocorticoids cause profound and varied metabolic effects. In addition, they modify the body's immune responses. Methylprednisolone is a potent anti-inflammatory steroid with greater anti-inflammatory potency than prednisolone and even less tendency than prednisolone to induce sodium and water retention.

She received more morphine at 6:50pm. The nurse will be giving her saline, metoprolol, Tylenol, Benadryl, Prevacid, and Norco for pain at 8:00pm. She may get insulin at that time if needed. The next dose of the IVIG is due at 10:00pm. 9:20pm sugar tested at 146, she is safe for now. Blood pressure is 131/52 and temperature is 98.2°.

9:50pm, here we go again. Another scheduled IVIG which we believe is helping her. The IVIG was complete at midnight. Another day is done.

January 6, 5:00am it is time for medication. Not much sleep around here. They increased the saline solution to bump up the sodium. Vitals test at: temperature 98.0°, blood pressure 133/48, sugar 201(uh-oh), hemoglobin at 7.0 (another more important uh-oh), platelets are 55 and sodium 130. Vein blood was drawn for cultures. The reduction in her arm swelling was just enough to permit a vein blood draw.

With the elbows propped up her arm movement was getting to a point where she could manage to get the suction tube to her mouth to help vacate her throat on her own. She still couldn't reach her face with her hand itself because the swelling was still big at the elbow making it hard to bend.

Testing and medicines kept her stabilized throughout the day. At 5:00pm the vitals were: sugar 115, temperature 97.4°, blood pressure 138/59, and heart rate at 84bpm. Robitussin and steroids were given at 5:35pm.

The night nurse shift occurred on schedule at 7:10pm. **I helped her roll my wife** so she could change the bedding. Sometimes it was more efficient to get involved. It also protected my wife from further stress because we didn't have to wait for enough help to show up to get the job done. The nurses seemed grateful for the extra help I could offer. 9:45pm medicine disbursement is: Primaxim antibiotic, stool softener, miralax, 30 units of long acting insulin, Prevacid, and Xanax. 11:15pm they started the third dose of this segment of the IVIG treatment. They were having trouble with the old delivery system machine, so they brought in a brand new one earlier in the day. They weren't sure how to calibrate it. They called in another nurse from a different part of the floor. He had good training on this machine and set it up for the procedure.

Chapter Five

ARE THINGS GETTING BETTER?

January 7 1:00am I woke up to an alarm going off. The IVIG was complete. I had fallen asleep. They took her blood pressure at 137/54. 4:50am more alarms are going off. The "new" feed control machine was on battery. It needed to be plugged in. All that science and we get tripped up on the basics (so much for a good night's sleep). A few minutes after 5:00am vitals are 133/49, temperature is 98°, and sugar 125. The nurse adjusted the pillows. This was a constant ritual to support my wife's elbows so she could use her arms.

8:00am the lung doctor thinks she is doing better. They can remove the oxygen tube that has been around the front of her nose. Her oxygen count has never gone below 98. Respiratory treatment showed up at this time. She will breathe into a mask full of vapor and medicine to keep her lungs clear. At 9:23am the hemoglobin count is reported at 6.7. They will have to give her **another unit of blood**. When is this going to stabilize?

About 9:45am I took a picture of her swollen arm. The movement was very difficult with the added weight of all the retained water. The hospital bracelet had been changed to allow for the swelling so as not to shut off her circulation. It had started to subside at the wrist area, but nearer the elbow it was still quite large making it hard to bend. Just the weight of that extra liquid made it hard to lift also, given the lack of muscle.

10:00am the team lead doctor came in to say they need to stabilize her before other medications can be considered for treatment. They feel she is improving enough to reduce their calls to an every other day basis, however. This is encouraging news, although progress seems to be ever so slow. It is difficult to know for sure, but these doctors may be withholding stories from us so as not to scare us. When they say they are going to come by every other day, I am assuming they have seen cases like this and now they feel it is only a matter of time to observe the healing process. **They may know they have gotten the patient through the worst of it.** Maybe I should have directly asked a question along those lines.

10:30am vitals are 141/50.

12:15pm the primary doctor is watching the infections and ordered a blood unit based on the last hemoglobin reading of 6.7. He told me he ordered an extra dose of steroids yesterday to try to shock the system into repair. I am going to look for improvements.

1:45pm a respiratory technician came in to give her breathing treatment. He approached her from her right side. The other side of the bed was crowded with a chair full of supplies. It was more advantageous to work from the other side next to the supply "tree". As he finished the 4 or 5 minute session, he removed the mask from her face and started to step away. Unknowingly, his foot had gotten tangled in the mass of tubing coming from the "tree" full of medicines, and saline, etc. **He stepped back and tripped backwards yanking the tubing from the med-port in her chest. My wife screamed. I yelled as I was**

observing from the other side of the bed. He was profoundly sorry and must have apologized 4 or more times over and over. The nurse heard the commotion outside in the hall. She came running in with another nurse. Now we were in a bad predicament. **The med-port may have been compromised and would have to be replaced.** How are we going to get a new unit of blood into her? She needs it badly. They looked at the port. It seemed alright. She will have to go for an x-ray to be sure it was still viable. At 2:10pm the gastro intestinal doctor came in to look at her stomach to find it much improved. 3:00pm she was transported for an x-ray of the port. It was still in good shape, but the **troubles were not over.** We still had to replace the cap on the port in order to administer the unit of blood and the medications. At 3:30pm the internal medicine doctor looked at the stomach. He said it looked good.

At 6:00pm they took the Foley out. Even though this is a more permanent type of catheter to empty the bladder, it cannot stay in too long for fear of infection. My wife **started taking shorter breaths** at this time. I noticed it in her speech. I made a mental note of it in case of future complications. I am so on edge when I sense these changes.

It was 6:45pm before the nurse got the port caps, of various sizes, from the pharmacy. He judged the size of the cap needed from the variety supplied by the pharmacy and put it into the port hole. The blood arrived at 7:00pm. The night nurse said she will administer the transfusion. Around 9:00pm vitals were taken. Sugar was 127, blood pressure 135/44. The nurse gave her Prevacid, stool softener, Norco, and Primaxim. It wasn't until 11:30pm the nurse showed up with another nurse to help her set up the unit of blood. I was getting very nervous about the long delay. This should have occurred mid-afternoon.

January 8, 12:15am I helped the nurse turn my wife. I noticed some strong purple bruising radiating out, to the front and back, from under both arms. The nurse couldn't explain it. Perhaps she is just prone to bruising because of all the medication and the absence of muscle to hold things together. The nurse said they will keep a watch on it. It indicated to me that they had possibly pulled her to the head of the bed by her arms when they adjusted her at some time.

1:15am, I took a picture of her lying in bed, swollen like a balloon. Her arms and fingers were puffed, her neck and face still swollen. The nurse call button unit was very close to her right hand so she could communicate the only way possible at this time.

About this time she said to me: **"Why don't I feel like I'm getting better?** We had an intimate conversation then, and she seemed to calm down.

At 2:55am the blood was finishing. It should be complete within the hour. The nurse did a bladder scan at 358ml and ordered the smaller catheter.

The infection in the old PEG tube incision has resisted medication. The nurses have to wear protective gowns and gloves now to avoid spreading the infection outside the room to other patients. I witnessed the nurse answering her cellphone, and operating her computer mouse while wearing her purple protective gloves and then continuing to work on the patient without changing gloves. (So much for hygiene!)

Now the nurse is trying to unplug the nose feed tube. It is supposed to be flushed after feeding and after medications. It is plugged now and won't flush right, **so the only way of feeding her is disabled. Now what are we going to do?**

(My wife is talking in short breaths again. This bothers me. Are the muscles controlling this function starting to breakdown?)

The feeding tube gets plugged because the "food" has dextrose in it. This sugary substance tends to dry into a rock hard barrier if it is not washed through right after completing the feed process. Also, the pills can't be given orally, of course, so they have to crush them in a very old press that looks like something from the long past. One would think, given the severity of this affliction, **they should have all liquid medicine** if it is required through the tube. The crushed pills do not dissolve thoroughly in water. As a result they are a constant menace to keeping the feed tube clean. The nurses seem reluctant to back down on the need for crushing, instead of requesting a liquid. Some obvious necessities seem overlooked in the day to day process, despite our modern age of medicine. **This crushing process seems so backward**.

The next nurse gets the result: a plugged feed tube. This nurse worked for a long time trying warm water, and cola syringes until finally it broke through. I am estimating it took her over a half an hour, poor thing! She worked very hard.

3:30am: lights out for now.

4:17am the lights are back on. They have to put in a straight catheter. The smaller size went easy. They extracted 500ml of urine.

6:45am the sugar count is 136.

I'm tired. I got little sleep. My wife is the sick one. I can imagine how she feels.

January 8th, 7:00am the night nurse worked on the feed tube. It is plugged again. The morning nurse was introduced to us. Sugar tested at 108 at 8:08am. My wife asked to be changed and cleaned up. They finished that chore by 8:30am. Blood pressure 152/67, temperature is 97.4°, oxygen reads at 100% (this has never been a problem).

At 9:30am I requested to see a head nurse. At 9:45am a customer service representative came in to listen to my concerns. I told her about the need for small catheters, the small veils for blood work, plugged feed tube, the respirator technician tripping on the tubing which delayed the blood transfusion, the mistreatment in ICU by physical therapy resulting in tearing her skin and subsequent infection. If it sounds like I am rambling on, I am. I was frustrated with all the back steps we were taking despite how hard my wife was trying. She will have a head nurse or a charge nurse discuss this with me. I need to get the message across.

10:15am occupational therapy came in. They sat her up, carefully. I was insistent they use caution considering all we went through the first time. They were very helpful. They had her rub her face, rub her hands together, and reach for things. They unsnarled her hair which was a good diversion from the effort of sitting. These exercises were extremely difficult for her since she still can barely operate her own suction tube without the assistance of pillows under her elbows.

11:00am the rheumatology doctor came in to say they can not consider any auto-immune therapy until the infections are stable. I expressed our fear of one of the choices called Rituximab.

11:35am she was taken to the x-ray lab for insertion of a new feed tube in her nose. When she came back they said the doctor was able to save the current tube by running a thin wire through under x-ray. This was good news. At least she had a minimum of discomfort this time. The negative observation is the possibility of shoving infected matter into the stomach.

When she got back the nurse gave her antibiotic, and Diflucan fungicidal. The platelet's count is 52, hemoglobin 8.5, and potassium is low.

1:05pm sugar count is 50. The nurse has to put up a new feed bag formula to bring up the sugar. It probably dropped during the overnight. She hadn't eaten for a while because the tube was plugged. At 2:45pm the infectious disease doctor said they may add another antibiotic. They are watching these infections closely. The concerns they are expressing are very bothersome to me. I will be paying close attention, myself.

4:00pm I left for home.

January 9th, 8:30am they are using a new antibiotic, Daptomycin. (Cubicin brand) used to treat bacterial infections of the skin and underlying tissues. I brought in some new Biotene Mouth Spray. She was running low on supply.

10:45pm her sugar is 151, temperature is 97.6°, blood pressure 141/53. The nurse gave her insulin, and pain medication.

3:15pm, she needs a catheter to relieve the bladder. Her hemoglobin is 8.3. It was 8.5 yesterday. That's not good. Potassium is 2.9, and sodium 132. Sugar tests out at 98(perfect). At 7:30pm we met the night nurse. My wife was able to pass her water on her own. This is a sign of things slowly returning, we hope. At 8:00pm the nurse gave her slow release insulin, Colace(stool softener), miralax, Norco, Prevacid,

and Motoprolol. At 9:15pm sugar is 112,
temperature 98.1°, and blood pressure 142/56.
The nurse gave her antibiotics at 9:44pm.

January 10, 6:30pm vitals taken were sugar 90,
temperature 97.0°, and her sonogram shows her
bladder containing 875ml, much too high. 7:50pm
the nurse and an aid tried to straight catheterize
her. I was in the room on my couch, giving them
their privacy. The nurse had her back to me,
hovering over the patient from just above waist
level. When they backed away from the bed I
asked if they were successful. The nurse said,
"No". I was surprised. It should have been easier.
I asked her if she used the smaller catheter from
the shelf.. She replied she didn't. She said she
used whatever the pharmacy sent up. I got pretty
firm when I scolded the nurse and pointed out
that there was a whole case of smaller catheters
on the shelf next to my couch. The other nurse
had ordered them so we would have the right one
available when needed. When we checked the
package of the one she was using from the
pharmacy, it was a #14. **I was horrified. This was**

supposed to be changed on her records since the incidents in the ICU. The nurse didn't notice any indications on her records to use a smaller size. I had to leave to take care of things at home, freshen up, and get some rest before returning the next day.

January 11, 11:55, sugar 87, vitals 155/48 blood pressure, 98.0°, hemoglobin 8.3, platelets 63, sodium 135, potassium 2.8(a little low). Her sodium seems to be stable lately. Sodium was the alarming reading that first brought us to the hospital. Hemoglobin seems to always be low. The doctors are stumped with the platelet count.

At 1:30pm the nurse had to catheterize her. This time she used the proper size. Her sonogram bladder scan was just under 900ml. The resulting plastic bag full of liquid reminded me of the shape of a loaf of deli meat you would find in a store. It is hard to imagine the body retaining that amount in the bladder. This was an indication to me of the lack of muscle in the body to perceive the sensations of the pressure from such a mass amount of liquid.

The team of doctors came in at 2:00pm. The team leader did the standard check on the muscle responses and reported she thought my wife was stronger.

The primary doctor stopped by at 2:30pm and said he is watching the stomach infection very closely.

4:45pm sugar count is 102.

8:31pm the night nurse is setting up saline. She just left to find some help to change my wife's bed and freshen her up for the evening. Two other nurses came in with her and they got the job done quickly. It is easier to roll the patient and hold her, while the other nurse rolls up the bedding and makes the replacement. Given the weight of the patient and the lack of the patient's ability to hold herself using the bedrail, the extra helpers make the job run smoothly.

9:15pm blood pressure 138/69, sugar is 160. She is getting medications of Metoprolol, Lantis (long acting insulin), Novalox (fast acting insulin 2 units). I sprayed her mouth with Biotene. She also needed some lip gloss. A little later the nurse tried to feed her through the nose tube. **It was plugged again**. She worked on it for over an hour, using warm water and cola. She wasn't going to give up. After all my complaining, I am sure the nurses did not want to be responsible for another screw up. She finally got the tube to flow through, a little after 11:00pm.

Right around midnight the bladder checked out at 845ml. The smaller catheter worked like a charm. I asked the nurse why they would choose a larger catheter when the smaller one is easier and less invasive to the patient. Her response was the time it takes to empty the bladder is longer with the smaller tube and they have so much to do. It seems the **comfort of the patient is secondary to their convenience in this case**.

I stayed the night.

January 12th, 8:00am, we met the day nurse. Medication was given at 8:50am: Metoprolol, Prevacid, and insulin. Vitals are: Potassium 3.1, hemoglobin 8.0 (why can't we find out why this keeps slipping?), platelets 60, and sugar 150.

9:40am the bladder scanned at nearly 800ml again. This isn't good, although the body might be getting rid of the liquid it is retaining. They had to catheterize her again. This time it was uneventful with the use of the smaller size.

The primary doctor showed up at 10:45am. He is watching our progress with special interest. He said he had her on a high dose of steroids for 3 days. He will note the progress. He will put her back on 60mg doses as before. He wants all of her infections cleared before he agrees with neurology to go forward with any other treatment. This doctor became personally helpful to us understanding how we were progressing.

January 13, 8:00am we have the same day nurse for the second day. Potassium is 2.9, hemoglobin 7.7 (here we go again) and platelets are 64. The IV dose of steroids is being set at 60mg once a day. The previous level was 60mg twice a day for 3 days. This must be what the primary doctor was referring to yesterday. 9:45am blood pressure is 127/58. Diflucan was being administered.

My wife hollered to me she was able to touch her nose. She was thrilled.

10:15am the primary doctor reassured us they are waiting for a couple more blood tests to be able to determine further treatments. I am feeling more comfortable with his constant attention and disclosures. It feels good to have someone show genuine personal concerns for your loved one. I felt somewhat of a bond with him. Sugar tested at 96 after he left.

At 11:00am the Zosyn antibiotic was complete. (Piperacillin and tazobactam are penicillin antibiotics that fight bacteria in the body. *Zosyn* is used to treat many different infections caused by bacteria, such as urinary tract infections, bone and joint infections, severe vaginal infections, stomach infections, skin infections, and pneumonia).

11:30am the bladder scan is 862, another big one. They will have to catheterize again. At 4:20 pm sugar is holding at 112.

1:05pm I took a picture of her sitting in the chair next to her bed. The lift team transferred her there. The pillows are carefully propped under each elbow so she can reach her face and utilize the suction tube on her own by her right hand. The nurse button unit is between her hands for best access. At this point she is able to muster up a courageous smile and to my delight, a wave of her left hand. She is trying to use the mouth spray by herself. Her hand strength isn't enough to push the plunger down at this time.

It is time for me to go home and regroup.

When I got home I checked my mail, took a shower, got some clothes ready for tomorrow, and warmed up some soup from one of the neighbors who is looking out for my welfare as this goes on.

January 14, 10:00am, we have a new day nurse, a well trained male. Hemoglobin is 7.4 (down again). 12:00 noon sugar is 41. 12:20pm the nurse gave her a dextrose solution to bring the sugar up. By 1:10pm the sugar came back and tested at 100. Vitals at 3:30pm are oxygen 97, temperature 97.9°, and blood pressure 114/42. At 6:00pm they check in at 124/44 blood pressure, temperature

98.5°, oxygen is 96(somewhat slipping but not a matter of alarm).

The night nurse is on duty now and had to attend to a bed change right away. The bladder muscles did not hold this time. As time is passing my wife seems to be able to hold the rail a little better each time they change her. She is developing a little more arm movement each day. With the help of the pillows under the elbows she can use the suction tube herself and blow her own nose.

The nurse gave her long acting insulin for the night. I can't figure the reasoning for this, since the sugar count was so low earlier in the day. About 11:50pm my wife was able to urinate about 100ml in the bed pan on her own, quite a contrast from earlier this evening.

I stayed the night.

January 15th, the night nurse took vitals at 6:30am. Sugar is 41 (Why did they even give her long acting insulin last night? It is always lower in the morning.). The bladder scan is 440ml which will require a catheterization again.

The day nurse arrived and started her shift at a little after 7am. At 8:45am blood pressure is 124/47 and 74bpm. She gave the patient prednisone, Prevacid, and Metoprolol. The respiratory treatment technician came by at 9:30am. The Speech Therapist evaluated the swallow at 9:45am. It is a busy morning so far. Blood pressure reading is 125/57.

2:24pm I took a picture of her left arm. Amazingly the swelling was gone. Her identification band was up to her elbow. Perhaps this is the result of the massive dose of steroids given two days ago. I felt we were turning a corner on a course to recovery. It had been two months since we started the journey at the clinic on November 13th.

Many things were going on from 2:30pm on. The Physicians Assistant for gastro came in to examine the stomach area. Then the infectious disease doctor came in to look at the stomach, also. We got a thumb's up. The infection seems to be clearing up. They will consider another try at a new PEG tube when all remains stable. The doctor looked at her muscle reflexes and thought she was getting stronger. The progress for the last couple of days seems to be positive, but at an ever-so-slow rate.

January 16th I arrived at 9:45am. My wife was waiting for the nurse to come in and bath her. No blood transfusion yet. 12:05pm the primary doctor will take another blood draw at 5pm to get a closer reading on the hemoglobin. He will contact the gastro doctor to see where his plans are for my wife. Potassium is 4.9, sodium 133, platelets 49, and hemoglobin is 6.9 (this is the basis for the decision to take the 5pm reading before another unit of blood is ordered).

Shortly after the primary doctor left the physical therapy team came in. They brought a special table that will help her to a standing position. They will transfer her to the table by sliding the bed material with her. The table has three straps on it. One is chest level, one is hip level, and the other is knee level. The base has a foot rest. This was very similar to a dolly used to move a refrigerator. The idea is to tilt this table to a near standing position to give the patient a sense of mobility and to encourage natural circulation in the body. There is a calibration on the underside that indicates the angle acquired. She was extremely nervous and scared, absolutely helpless if something should go wrong. They strapped her in. As they cranked the table forward she asked them to wait until she got the courage to go further. The next crank produced and angle of about 55°. To her it felt like she was straight up. She asked them not to go any further. It is most likely the kind of feeling one gets on a roller coaster on that first straight down drop. When you observe that from the side, one can see there is a safe angle for the drop. At this point they wheeled the standing table, with her feet resting on the provided lip at the bottom, toward the window. This is the first real look she had gotten to see the outside world in nearly two months. I took a picture of her. Her right arm was still swollen, although I could see a gradual taper in the forearm. **She gave me a courageous wave with her left arm as she "stood" there in her knitted yellow hospital socks.**

At 1:00pm the bladder reading is 900. We need

a catheter again. When she was relieved of the water, they asked her if she would try sitting in the chair. She is always agreeable, since she knows this is the best way to fight for improvement.. At 1:28pm the lift team came in and put her in the chair.

It is 3:30 and the nurse is changing the dressing and cleaning around the med-port. When that was complete she wanted to be returned to bed. She had spent over two hours in the chair.

January 17th the morning nurse is in. The primary doctor came in at 9:45am and said he chose not to give her blood this time. He wanted to see if the body can revive the count on its own. To our surprise the hemoglobin count was 8.4. This is a good indication that things might be coming back. The potassium was 2.8 (normally, your blood potassium level is 3.6 to 5.2), and platelet count is 96. He will prescribe magnesium and maybe potassium to bring that count up. 12:15pm the sugar count is 108, another good sign. By 5:00pm the sugar had only risen to 113. Of course, the diet they maintain her on helps this area. Her temperature is 97.9°, blood pressure is 128/61 and oxygen is 100%.

5:45pm they changed the cap on the med-port which must be done every 7 days to prevent infection. 6:05pm she is getting more meds. The nurse's shift changed at the 7:00 hour. By 9:50pm she needed long acting insulin to get through the night. She also got Metoprolol, Prevacid, and antibiotics. By 10:25pm her blood sugar count was 137. I stayed the night.

Chapter Six

THINGS ARE STARTING TO CHANGE

It is 4:00am on the morning of January 18th, and they woke my wife up to give her more medication and draw blood samples. At 6:45am the blood pressure was taken and was 110/50. The bladder scan is 330ml so they had to use the catheter and drew 400ml. They said sometimes the scan isn't exact. That is why they don't like to go over 250ml.

7:24am **hemoglobin is reported at 6.0 (whoa- another scare).** Potassium is 3.9, magnesium 2.1, platelets 64, and sodium 132. Sodium was the first reading that brought us to the hospital scene, and now it seems to be the only count that is holding. The other numbers are not good.

The day nurse came in a little late, 7:41am. She took blood samples and reported **hemoglobin at 7.0, very confusing**. Perhaps I heard the first report wrong. Not surprising, with all the interrupted sleep. I will still have to be ready for the next news of a necessary transfusion.

I have been sleeping on the couch covered with a foam mattress topper provided by a caring nurse. I am told they appreciate my being there. My observations take some pressure off them. They can't remember each patients every item. They read from the computer screen and ask the patient, also. The more questions they ask the better cross check they have. Taking notes has been **my** best tool so far.

At 9:22am I took a picture of my wife using her own suction tube with her right hand. Although **the swelling has returned in her arms** she still has use of both her arms to the elbows at this point, as long as we continue to prop each one with a pillow. It seems we get 2 steps forward and 1 step back, but, it is progress of a sort.

Physical training team arrived at 10:00am with the table we tried two days ago. She was anxious to do this one again. This time she knew what to expect. They used the "slide-sheet" to transfer her. They put the 3 straps around her, as before, and cranked her up to 50°, and asked her if she was comfortable. I took pictures of this very proud moment. They then went to 55°, and after resting a bit, went to 60°. It was then she got a little nervous and asked them to stop there. This is still a great accomplishment because it is instilling an incentive to get up and get better, and, although she can't stand on her own, it is putting her body in the right position for better circulation.

It's 10:42am and Physical training is leaving. This was a good session. The blood pressure reading is 102/48. They are going to hold off on the Metoprolol. She is getting some potassium.

At 1:00pm the nurse is trying to balance the schedule of blood draws and administering medication. We had been expressing a need for some rest. After all, just look at this morning's schedule. Since 4:00 this morning they just put her through a full day of "work", and she is a sick person. She needs some solid sleep.

2:00pm the primary doctor held off drawing more blood after hearing our concerns. He decided to wait until morning. I left at 3:30pm today and left her in the hands of the staff.

I arrived at 9:45 the next morning of January 19. Hemoglobin is the first count I am asking for. It is 6.8, (not good, again). Blood pressure is 123/49. At 12:25pm her sugar is 103.

She was able to relieve her bladder on her own around 4:15pm. The 5:00pm report for hemoglobin is 7.0. Despite reaching the border line on the up side, the doctor ordered another unit of blood anyway, rather than take any chances with this close count. At 7:25pm they started the transfusion. The nurses were changing shifts at the same time.

My wife was able to empty her bladder at 8:20pm. Sugar is 134 at 9:15pm.

Medications at 10:45pm are Prevacid, Lantis (long acting insulin), and Metoprolol. They chose not to give her stool softener or Miralax at this time.

The transfusion was still trickling at 11:25pm and was scheduled to come down by 11:30pm for freshness purposes. It was taken down at 11:50pm and appeared to me to be only 50% used up. For some reason it didn't seem to enter the body the way others did.

It's 2:00am on January 20th morning, and she emptied her bladder on her own, again. They changed her gown and bedding. 4:15am she called for the nurse. The hose in the leg pump was cutting into her ankle. This pump periodically inflates sleeves that are placed around the calves of her legs, to encourage circulation and eliminate blood clots. At 6:30am she emptied her bladder again. The bladder scan showed 262ml left, but **they were happy things are happening in a natural way**. Sugar tested at 77. The lab report was in for hemoglobin at 7.3, not much of a boost from the roughly "half" unit of blood earlier. I think my observation was right. She didn't get that entire last unit.

It is the morning shift of January 20 and the daytime nurse is on the job. 8:10am a team doctor came in early and tested her responses. The doctor said she seemed stronger. 8:20am she requested a bed pan,(false alarm). 9:30am, the vitals are 133/57 blood pressure, and temperature 97.7°. 10 until 10:40am: was potty time.

The respiratory team came in at 10:45am and gave her breathing treatment with the mask until 11:00am. Immediately following I took the time to execute my own version of physical therapy. I started with her arms, slowly moving them in various directions to rekindle range of motion and muscle memory. I would ask her for a pain report as I reached certain levels. I don't want to cause damage, just tone the muscles gradually. I used much the same technique with the legs, slowly moving them in various ups and downs within the range restricted by the slightest pain. My hope is to gradually expand on that range and encourage the muscles to respond and rebuild.

At 2:30pm the internal medicine doctor came in to discuss the future. Given the fact that the PEG tube produced a previous infection, he felt they will wait on the chemotherapy Methotraxate, but the steroids will remain at current level until the new PEG tube is redone. **He will come back in a week** to see how she tolerates a new PEG tube. If no infection develops this time, we can go ahead with the chemo treatment. Otherwise, she is ready now. So, here we are: one step forward two steps back, **playing a waiting game.**

January 21st, 7:10am the morning nurse has checked in. She informed us **the new PEG tube operation is scheduled for today,** (That was fast news!). Hemoglobin is 9.5(yippee!), potassium is 2.9. 7:32am, she made quick order of the bed pan, relieving the bladder on her own. Blood pressure at 9:11am is 137/65. 10:00am I saw a good opportunity to give her my "version" of Physical Therapy as we did yesterday. I have to take those opportunities when I can. Her schedule is very busy.

The lift team came in at 1:30pm and sat her up in the chair for awhile. The nurse had informed us the new PEG tube operation will probably be done around 2:00pm. Things don't always happen as planned. The transport team finally came in about 3:45pm to wheel her to the operating floor. We arrived at the operation room at 4:00pm. I waited. At 5:00pm a nurse came in to say all went well. **The new tube was in**.

Back at the room the evening nurse took blood pressure reading at 7:00pm. It was 148/64. It was just a little higher than it has been, but not bad after a recent procedure. 9:20pm, more medication: Metoprolol, antibiotics, and morphine for the pain around the new incision of the new PEG tube, but now they can administer it through the PEG tube. This time around I insisted that she always wear a stomach binder. The binder was about a 10 inch wide elastic and cotton strip that wrapped completely around the waist. It doubled up in the front and secured itself with a "Velcro" strip at the end that caught on the material of the binder at any needed point.

I stayed the night to keep an eye on things.

January 22nd, 2:45am she woke up and requested the bed pan. That went very well. She says she feels more secure with the abdominal binder on. It's a good thing I saved the old one from ICU. The new one I asked for never showed up ("go figure!"). I have learned to stay one step ahead of these people lately.

3:10am they are giving her more medications. She is getting morphine, Norco, antibiotics, and pedialight. At 8:05am my wife and I decided to forgo the lift team to avoid further trauma to her stomach for this time. We discussed how **this was done too soon the first time she had a PEG tube**. One day of rest isn't going to mess up the long range goal of getting her active and well. Besides, this muscle thing is more than **they** are accustomed to dealing with in my estimation.

She got more medications consisting of Prevacid, steroids, miralax, cranberry juice, and antibiotics. Sugar tested at 195. Hemoglobin is reported at 7.5, platelets at 98, and sodium 135. It is so reassuring to get medication through the new PEG-tube now and not worry about it plugging up, although this can also happen to this larger opening if they are not careful. She is also able to spray her own throat with the Biotene as needed. and can apply her lip gloss.

It's 7:00pm and the night nurse came in to introduce herself. At 7:20pm the nurse gave my wife a much appreciated bath. The nurse decided to treat her favorite "customer". We would get side stories from the nurses, regarding other patients. One they told us was the guy down the hall insisting on male nurses because women are "stupid". He wasn't making his stay any more pleasant that way. My wife didn't push the nurses or ask for much. They all seemed to appreciate her. Following the bath she did a bladder scan and had to use the catheter. A little after 9:00pm sugar is 127, blood pressure is 118/47 and temperature is 98.0°. A bladder scan at this time is only 99. More meds at 10:00pm: Metoprolol, and Prevacid. These vitals are much more normal.

January 23, 2:45am she relieved her bladder, but a check up bladder scan reveals over 400ml left. They will hold off for awhile to see if she goes again and relieves more on her own. 6:00am, blood pressure is 135/47. Sugar is 164. They will probably give her a shot of insulin.

It is now 7:00am on January 23rd, and the morning nurse is drawing blood for testing. She gave my wife some Robitussin. The respiratory tech came in at 8:20am to give her another breathing treatment. The individual who tripped on her line was never assigned to her again. These treatments are quite regular now, but welcomed because it reassures us that we are more likely to avoid the dreaded pneumonia.

My sister and brother-in-law came in to visit at 10:00am. Hemoglobin is reported down to 7.3. Here we go again.

I went home while my wife had family to watch over her.

January 24, 9:45am I arrived and met the day nurse. 11:42am the sugar is 148, potassium 3.3, magnesium is 1.4, platelets 119, and hemoglobin is 7.4. I am glad there is a digital clock on the wall so I can record everything at the time that they use. 2:00pm blood pressure is 134/65 and temperature is 98.0°. 5:10pm, sugar is 205. She is going to need a shot of insulin. Blood pressure is

135/43. I left for home and dinner. Things seemed under control.

January 25, I arrived at 10:45am. Hemoglobin is 7.5 (appears to be holding, though not very high). The bed pan was used at 2:30pm.

The primary doctor came in at 2:55pm to say she is doing much better. This is good to hear, but the progress is so slow, it tries one's patience. Lately we seem to be zeroing in on numbers, trying to stabilize all the vital counts. It isn't like waiting for someone to recover from a cold or the flu.

I took the time to do more physical therapy on her legs, to give us every advantage. I then left for home. Things were appearing to be more on a routine now.

January 26th, 10:00am, I arrived and asked for the vital counts. Potassium is 3.1, hemoglobin is up to 7.9 . I started physical therapy on her legs. **She can do her self exercises on her arms now.**

Her legs are still slow in coming around. Just before noon her sugar count is 160. She managed to use the bed pan shortly after noon. Things are starting to function on their own.

Occupational therapy came in at 3:00pm and worked on her arms. They covered the simple actions of brushing her hair, and washing her face and hands. This gives her a target for exercise.

The primary doctor came in at 4:15pm and gave her a check up. "The lungs sound good". She required another bedpan at 4:45pm. A respiratory treatment was given at 7:30pm. They really want to avoid pneumonia. We don't want to give in now that we have come so far.

January 27th, 2:00am was bedpan time. Two nurses rushed in to get to her in time. Since we have been here for such a long stay the nurses are all aware of her needs and are very willing to help. She gives them very little trouble during the normal routines of the day. She is also so very cooperative when it comes to the various technical duties they want her to perform. We all have to go in the middle of the night at times. I made some personal observations for myself. Someday it might be my turn in a hospital and I want to know how to behave. I would like to get the caring treatment she gets because of her behavior.

6:15am came quickly and the nurse gave her another bladder scan. It is time to use the bedpan again. Some of the natural functions are becoming a little more regular now.

8:10am one of the team doctors came in for a check on her. **He noticed some swelling returning on her left arm**. He wants to do a sonogram to eliminate possible blood clots. Another respiratory technician visited at 8:50am. At 9:50am the counts are reported as potassium 2.9, hemoglobin 7.8, and blood pressure 143/55. Blood pressure at 2:10pm is 131/62. I will mention at this point that I took care of emptying the suction receptacle as often as I could. This unit hung on the wall with a plastic cup that received the rinse water and the mucus from her throat tube. It was hooked to the vacuum line in the wall. I would rinse it and set it up so she had the maximum results she needed. I haven't mentioned the suctioning enough because it is a constant way of life for her at this point, as is the Biotene spray, and I got into the cleaning part of it like a "day at work". I tend to forget the different ways I pitched in to help. I also would fold and organize the blankets, sheets, towels, and pillow cases the nurses constantly threw all over the room. This also was on-going. Every thing they used was getting misplaced until I came up with an organized system. This system paid back sometimes at the most urgent moments when they were trying to make my wife comfortable.

At 2:35pm the main team neurologist doctor examined her, having her push up and down on her feet, and moving her legs and arms. Pulling and pushing for strength. The doctor checked her eye movement, fingers and hand motions. The neurologist is very impressed with her muscular improvements, and was particularly thorough this time. She also acknowledged we would be starting the next session of IVIG today. This would indicate my wife is clear of any infections that would otherwise prevent this.

The rheumatologist came in at 3:00pm and said things are looking good. If tests stay clean we will be able to start Methotrexate next week. Physical therapy showed up at the same time. When the doctor left the therapist began his session and tried an exercise on her legs. He pushed the sheets up to her knees to expose her lower legs and the feet in their yellow socks. **He asked her to try to spread her legs sideways toward the edges of the bed**. He had to help her to give her the idea. She then scuffed them away from each other on her own, ever so slightly, but it was progress. He then set them apart and asked her to bring them together. Again she scuffed the sheet as she dragged them together a couple of inches each. This was such a thrill to watch because until now we hadn't seen any indication of strength in that area. We only were able to get her to wiggle her toes and bring her feet back and forth like stepping on a gas peddle in the car. What a thrill to watch. I took a brief movie of this moment.

It's 5:45pm and they are giving her Tylenol, and Benadryl as required before the IVIG. At 7:00pm they set up the blood pressure monitor and set up the IVIG. The IVIG was turned on at 7:10pm and finished at 8:40pm. The new protocol for this procedure is a faster step-up timing now. The first IVIG sessions were much slower release. I was wondering: "**Are they learning as they go along,** because this affliction is so rare?"

The respiratory technician came in again at 8:45pm for another session.

January 28th, things are getting to be pretty repetitive. It would be nice to get out of here and continue at home. The problems of course are the lack of her mobility and the special care still needed. Other than bed pan reports, medicine sessions, and the daily therapy, there isn't much new today. Hemoglobin is 7.3 to start the morning. Sugar is 168. I left for the afternoon at 2:00pm. I am glad she is still there in case of relapse. **I know we have to be patient.**

I arrived at 9:00am, the morning of January 29. The nurse gave me the hemoglobin count right away. It was 7.6. He was aware of my concerns, and had that count ready when I walked into the room. At 1:30pm the team's lead doctor and another came in to say **they are ready to start Methotrexate** on Monday.

Bedpan duties came at 2:45pm. A short while later flowers from our son arrived. Certainly these were a welcomed piece of cheer. It really feels good seeing flowers arrive, instead of machines and medicine.

I performed some physical therapy on her legs and arms and left for home about 3:45pm. She was quite comfortable.

It's January 30th, Saturday, and another day of routines. I arrived at 10:30am, growing more confident every day. At 11:30am the lift team came in to move her to the chair located near the window. The nurse gave me the vitals report just before I took a lunch break to the hospital cafeteria. Blood pressure is 123/58 and hemoglobin is 7.3. I got back to the room with my sandwich as quickly as I could, and spent some time with my wife while she relaxed in her chair.

We sat for about an hour. As we gazed out the window we were treated to a pleasant sight of a clipper ship replica arriving in the bay. This weekend is the festival celebrating a local legend. We were told it is a big tradition here. We would be able to watch it unfold from our room. More yachts and boats filled the bay area, packing in tightly. A very large yacht appeared, boasting three decks. It looked out of place. We speculated on who would own such a boat. This was refreshing time spent. I am sure it took her mind off the grueling schedule we have been through.

It's January 31^{st,} Sunday morning, and I am awake at 5:30am to the sound of the nurses getting the vitals' numbers. Blood pressure is 128/51 and sugar is 100 Potassium was reported as "low", and hemoglobin is 7.3. She is in pretty good shape here.

The new day nurse came in on time this morning and suggested that this would be a good day to try something new. She thought we could get the lift team to **transfer my wife to a wheel**

chair so that we could take a tour outside the room. Can you imagine the thrill of such a suggestion? She was finally going to get out of the confines of the four walls of a hospital room and experience life. It must have been almost a feeling of getting released from a prison sentence.

About 8:30 the cleaning lady made her regular rounds and brought me a surprise cup of coffee. How nice of her. You get to make so many friends during a long ordeal like this. We shared some of her personal stories for a moment. She came from a substantial employment background. This job was a means of survival for the present.

12:05pm, the lift team arrived to transfer her to a wheel chair. The excitement was apparent. The nurse was anxious. Word was getting around. My wife is quite well known by now. At 12:11pm we headed for the door. As we made the turn and headed toward the nurses station, she was greeted to a round of applause. **I got tears in my eyes.**

. Within 10 minutes I was able to take a picture of her sitting in the wheel chair at the main entrance of the hospital enjoying her first breath of fresh air in two months. We rolled the chair to the garden area between the hospital wings. We spent a few moments reminiscing how far we have come. We then took off down the sidewalks, into the cafeteria, through the halls that I have seen so many times, so she could get a feeling for the places I have travelled while visiting her each day. We returned to the room within the hour. The nurse took vitals of blood pressure at 128/55 and a heart rate of 72 bpm. Temperature is 98.0° at 1:15pm.

Sugar count at 4:02pm is 155. The bedpan was needed at 4:30pm. I headed for home about 4:45pm.

Chapter Seven

IT IS FEBRUARY ALREADY

February 1st, I arrived about 9:10am. The nurse reported her hemoglobin was down to near 7.0. Potassium was low too. (Here we go again!) 10:20am is medication time. Vitals are recorded as 98.0°, and blood pressure is 136/68.

1:00pm the team doctors came in for their routine check-up. They did the muscle check on the arms and legs and feet. The hands are checked with spread fingers that the doctor squeezes to check resistance. They give all these checks a number to compare next time.

It is just before 2:00pm and an Occupational Therapy technician came in to get her to sit up. It was painful getting into the sitting position. Once she was there the tech let her sit without holding on to her. She was nearby, but wanted my wife to believe that she could sit and balance herself. It was a major accomplishment. I took a picture. She was proud.

At 2:20pm we had a visitor from a rehab center. She wanted to discuss the future arrangements that will be necessary when my wife is ready to leave the general hospital environment. I listened carefully to obtain as much information as I could. I wasn't convinced that we were going anywhere very soon. Someone from administration conveys the progress and tries to help the patient through the transition. This only proves to me that the general feeling going on here is that she is getting better. We have, by this time, stopped propping the pillows under her elbows. She prefers working her arms as much as she can to build strength. The swelling has gone away and the arms are much more lightweight. She is able to suction her own throat.

3:56pm is bath time today. They have special wipes for the body, and a shampoo cap which is put over the hair with the special shampoo in it. After it is messaged into the hair it is merely dried off with a towel. She is beginning to lose her hair.

There is a bald spot at the crown where her head rubs as they slide her up to the top of the bed. Her neck muscles don't hold her head up, so it drags there.

A new nightgown and a bedding change is due. 5:24pm, sugar is 164. She got a shot of insulin. At 9:44pm sugar tested at 136.

10:50pm medicines included mouthwash, Heparin (blood thinner), Prevacid, and Metoprolol for blood pressure. Monday is to be the start of the Methotrexate dosage. She is to take 1 tablet per week at a dosage of 2.5mg. This will be accompanied by Folate (folic acid). We are told the normal folic acid level is depleted by the Methotrexate.

February 2nd. The day nurse is reporting a hemoglobin count of 6.8, (Oh no! I know what that means!). Very soon I will be hearing about another scheduled blood transfusion.

8:45am she is given medicines including Prevacid, folic acid, prednisone, potassium and Metoprolol.

The lift team came at 11:00am to put my wife in a wheel chair. **For the second time** in the last few days **we were able to take a ride outside the room** and through the halls. We went down to the back section where the restaurant is and spent time at the outdoor tables for a lunch hour for me. This was a refreshing time spent.

About 1:00pm we were back in the room for medication. She received something to reduce the risk of blood clots.

February 3rd, 3:28pm the primary doctor said he will talk to rheumatology about the possibility of receiving the Methotrexate subcutaneously. This will avoid crushing the pill and possibly clogging the PEG tube. They respect the toxicity of this drug and want as little risk of spillage and personal contamination.

At 6:30pm I worked on her legs. My physical therapy is extra effort to hopefully advance the healing process. I took a picture of her leg, after the therapy, to indicate the progress of her being able to lift it off the surface of the bed. I placed a pillow behind the knee to give it elevation and then took a video of the leg **as she lifted the heal approximately 1" off the bed**. What amazing progress!

6:45pm blood pressure is 149/79, sugar is 137. At 9:35pm blood pressure is 138/63 and sugar 96. It is pretty interesting how these numbers can fluctuate. It is no wonder we are having trouble stabilizing everything. At 9:58pm we called for a bed pan. By 10:03pm I had to do the duty myself. We were running out of time (and patience), and the moment was urgent. Night medication consisted of colace, miralax and a bowel wash. We were told a colonoscopy is finally scheduled tomorrow to rule out GI bleeding. With the special medication for the bowel, the bedpan was hourly all night long. The nurses got a workout.

I stayed the night to be ready for the next big day.

February 4th, the morning readings are Hemoglobin 8.2, and potassium is 3.0. We are told the colonoscopy is scheduled for 1:30pm.

The 8:45am reading for sugar is 74, and blood pressure 127/57. 10:05am another bedpan session. At noon the sugar is 98. 1:53pm blood pressure is 129/58 and temperature is taken at 97.8°. We are ready for the trip to the operating room for the colonoscopy.

Things don't always go as planned. By the time we got down to the preparation room it was after 2:30pm. This stop at the room included taking more vitals and securing a tape to her forehead that is heat sensitive and indicates her temperature by a glowing color on the calibration printed on it (how modern!). I waited in that room after they wheeled her out in her bed. When they brought her back to the room for recovery she was very sleepy. The doctor came in shortly to tell us that he found **no indications of bleeding, or cancer**. He found diverticulosis, but we were aware of that condition from other colonoscopies she had done in years past. When the doctor left the room I saw tears welling up in her eyes. I said this was good news and asked what she was crying about. She told me she was so afraid she had cancer. I said I wished she would have shared those fears with me before. I could have told her that the bone marrow biopsy ruled that out a month ago.

What a tender moment!

I was aware now that she has been trying to second guess her illness, in case we were protecting her from the "truth", as she suspected it to be. It is hard to guess what goes on in my loved one's mind, but, with patience, I have to be ready to address her fears. She also wasn't able to remember a lot about her time in ICU. **I guess I didn't even realize how sick she was then.**

After about a half hour in the recovery room a nurse came in to give her a final check, and made arrangements for transport to take her back to her room. Once back in the room and being assured she was comfortable, I left for home just as the nurse shift was making there exchange, around the 7:00pm hour.

February 5th, hemoglobin is holding at 8.2. A couple of our friends came by to visit. It seems we are getting more visitors as things seem to be making a turn for the better, and she has more strength for visitors. At 1:30pm she left for speech therapy evaluation. They wanted to watch her swallow on the x-ray and evaluate her progress. The message coming back afterward was she is "getting better". It is 2:30pm and we have more company. Her brother and his wife came in to see her. They brought her a small planter.

The team lead doctor came by at 3:30pm to do a muscle study. She felt my wife was improving. I asked her to witness something my wife and I were practicing. I was working on getting my wife to reach upward for a pill box I was holding. The purpose was to get her to lift her elbow off the bed while reaching straight up. (We did it the night before, and with a shaking hand she was able to just touch the pill box.) The doctor watched as I prepared this demonstration. **As I held the pill box above her hand, she reached up and grabbed the pill box right out of my hand.** I was so surprised the doctor laughed. I asked my wife how she came to do that. She said she practiced all night. What a "trooper"!

The primary doctor came in at 4:30pm. She will

check on the stomach medication that was suggested by the gastro-intestinal doctor. She will also prescribe the Methotrexate to be administered subcutaneously on Monday. This will eliminate the need to crush this toxic pill that would have to be given through the PEG tube.

At 5:13pm the medicine is guaifenesin, insulin, and the antibiotic. Meparin started on February 3rd, ordered by rheumatology. At 8:33pm the medicine is Metoprolol, Prevacid, and Miralax. Blood pressure is 141/60, with 98bpm.

February 6 the morning nurse is reporting hemoglobin at 7.8. At 9:38am the medicines are Metoprolol, folic acid, Prevacid, and Prednisone 40mg, potassium, and a protein shot. She got no Miralax, and no Colace. 12:30pm the sugar tested at 136, and her temperature is 98.1°.

February 7th, I arrived at 10:30am to find my wife already sitting in her chair. I checked the hemoglobin count right away with the day nurse. It is 7.9. The nurse tells me the potassium count is low again. I keep trying to think of reasons why these counts keep fluctuating. I think the doctors are just tweaking all of this stuff with medicines, and waiting for the body to naturally "kick-in" and take over to bring things back to normal. The body presents itself to me as something truly amazing. When it goes out of sync our medical experts are still guessing at things to do to make it better, but each medicine seems to produce a reaction to offset something else. At least we have these medicines to help the system as it struggles against the odds.

I proceeded to set my wife up with her laptop. She is starting to show a lot of interest in doing work remotely on the computer for her brother's business. This is giving her a sense of being needed. The incentive is a great motivator to help her achieve more goals. She also demonstrated to me her improved ability to write. A sure improvement from the day in ICU when she put her "X" on the permission form for me. All these things are great signs we are moving in a positive direction. She remained in the chair for a long time. She finally requested to be moved back to the bed about 2:00pm. Although the long duration in the chair is encouraging, it is still a difficult session when a person cannot move around substantially to get a better position and work out the aches that build in the body from staying in one place too long. She is continually fighting bed sores. Being on her back so long, she developed bed sores. One of the medicines the nurses are always looking for is "Triple Butt Paste". It comes in a white plastic jar with a twist off cap that comes sealed with a piece of red paper tape across the top. It is easy to spot, but always absent mindedly set aside. It is a thick white cream that "sticks" to the wounded area to offer healing properties for a longer duration than other salves. I try to keep tract of this item for them. They use a lot of it

At 3:00pm the gastro doctor came by to report things are looking good from his perspective. He is following this PEG tube a little closer this time. He appreciated our use of the binder, given the results of the first one.

At 7:00pm the nurses took advantage of the shift change to help each other clean and change the Med-port set up. This is a careful procedure that requires particular attention to cleanliness. It is much more reassuring with assistance. Using alcohol swabs and a special square bandage, one nurse manipulates removing the old dressing and handing things back and forth to the other nurse as an assistant. One person could do this, but they want to be so sure that they don't drop anything on the open area after cleaning it properly. With hands basically freed from the old pieces, the main attendant can concentrate on a good clean fit and seal for the new dressing. Infection is their big concern.

At 9:00pm the basic medications were given. Sugar tested at 133. The night nurse put in the new port cap in the Med-port. She used heparin to clear the line. She also gave her the nighttime dose of miralax. We began talking about the little rest she is afforded with all this medicine and testing. There must be a way to coordinate their schedules. More sleep should equal better healing at this stage of her progress.

Things are getting a little more comfortable now. We spend time in the room together watching favorite TV shows. We pass the time with some exercises. I am constantly wiping down the tables and serving tray. I am still cleaning the accumulator tank for the suction tube so it doesn't get clogged and gives her maximum suction to keep her throat clear. I also continue to organize the sheets, and blankets, etc.

February 8th, Monday, the morning nurse looked up the hemoglobin report for me. It is 7.8. I continue to worry about that number. One of the neurologists came by at 8:30 to give her a pre-exam before the team comes in. She checked all the muscle movements in the routine and said things are looking pretty good.

At 9:15am the blood pressure is 125/56 and temperature is 98.7°. Medication is a little different this morning. This is Monday morning. They have designated this day as the Methotrexate day. So, she will be getting a subcutaneous dose of Methotrexate this time. She also has to have folic acid with it to balance the effects on her system. The Prevacid and Carafate help to offset the harshness of the medications. And, she gets her usual dose of

Metoprolol.

It's 11:30am and **the speech therapist wants to try a stimulator**. She explains that it is taped under the chin and has electrodes that are connected to a battery pack. The controller sends a vibrating type "shock" signal to the electrodes to encourage the throat muscles to "remember" how to contract. In the meanwhile she is leaving an instruction sheet with specific throat exercises which include dramatic swallowing attempts and singing "Ah-eeee" to use and build the throat muscles.

When the primary doctor arrived at noon we told her about the stimulator idea. She thought this should be ok, and will discuss it with the speech therapist. We also asked her to think about getting a sleep schedule established to get more rest and encourage healing. She thought this is a good idea and will discuss it with the nurses at the station.

Since the Methotrexate is being administered with a needle subcutaneously, it requires two special nurses from oncology, to administer it safely. They arrived at 2:00pm to give the shot.

Great care is taken to give the shot entirely, with no spills or contamination to anyone or anything in the room. They are wearing special, thicker gowns and gloves for their own protection. My wife and I are instructed that the toxic period following this moment will expire every Wednesday following. The 48 hours in between are when we should avoid contacting any of her body fluids directly. **I and the nurses will have to wear thicker gowns during this period.**

It's 2:30pm and she requested to go to her chair. The lift team was called. About an hour later we got her back into her bed. I set her up with her computer so she could do some "human" things. She looked quite happy being set up like an office. This was great for her well being. Judging by the look on her face, she was set. When she was comfortable, I took a picture of her sitting there and then left for home a little after 3:30pm.

February 9, I arrived at 11:10am and checked in with the day nurse. The hemoglobin count was up to 8.3. Perhaps this is due to the new sleep cycle she experienced last night. I hope so. The primary doctor instructed the crew at the nurse's station to post a, "do not disturb between 12 and 5am", sign on the door. I did not get a current potassium count. My wife was in the chair already, and looked somewhat refreshed and rested. I had to take a picture of her with a big smile on her face. After being in the hospital for over 2 months, this rest idea is coming at just the right time. This kind of schedule should give her a feeling like being home, almost like getting a natural night's sleep. This is the time to make progress toward recovery. I think this will be a key element to her recovery.

The primary doctor came by again today, at 12:30pm, for her final check. She informed us she was making a career move to California where she had a sibling. We are certainly going to miss her. She had the ultimate concern for my wife.

It's 4:15pm and the blood pressure is 129/55, with heart rate at 82bpm. Carafate and antibiotics are given today at 5:30pm.

The night nurse did her vitals' check at 8:55pm. Sugar is 127, blood pressure is 127/50, and temperature is 97.0°. 9:00pm medicines are Carafate, Heparin, and Prevacid. Although we had an opportunity to get another decent night's rest, we were interrupted by a malfunctioning feeding machine at 1:30am. Damn! At 2:45am we had to call for a bed pan anyway. She still is unable to navigate on her own legs to use the bathroom, although, she is getting more movement in her legs everyday. (So much for well-laid resting plans)

6:30am came fast. Blood pressure reading is 116/59, and medication is being given.

It is now 9:00am on the morning of February 10, time for more medication: Prevacid, Metoprolol, folic acid, Prednisone, potassium, and Carafate. She did not take Colace, Miralax or insulin.

Someone left a fresh cup of coffee for me. I don't even know who to thank.

At 9:30am a new primary doctor came by to say he has been watching this case very carefully. This doctor had been assigned to us before.

When the other primary doctor moved on to California, he took the return assignment. He assured us he would do everything he could to help us. He said he checked on the hemoglobin count. It was 8.2 today. He remembered this being a concerning number in the past.

At 10:00am a team doctor came in to give her a muscle evaluation. At 10:30am I worked on her leg exercises. I noted a severe scaling on the bottom of her feet. I had to peel away the **thick crusted skin** and apply cream to soften it up. All this time in bed dried the skin to a crust resembling a leather bottom slipper. It came off in large thick pieces, much like a shell of a lobster tail. I had never seen anything like this.

12:00pm is time for more routine medicines, along with Heparin, and Robitussin. By 2:00pm she is ready for a trip to her chair. First they took her blood pressure at 129/57, with temperature of 98.7°.

While transferring to the chair via the sling, the lift team is able to get a weight reading. This is something new to us. She weighs in at 127lbs today. As a note of reference, she was normally

155lbs before being hospitalized. She was 208lbs upon arriving at the General Hospital on December 11th. Now that she has shed all the extra fluid, **she is a much lighter person with little muscle matter.**

The dietician came by at 2:45pm with a suggestion for **bolus feeding**. This would require pouring a prepared liquid food compound directly into the PEG tube through a funnel-like apparatus that would allow the food to enter the stomach by gravity. This takes an administrator's time, but is beneficial in developing a feeding cycle, as apposed to a slow steady stream of nutrients. **This cycle would bring the body back to familiar rhythms.**

2:50pm, Physical Therapy team is in the room with a machine designed to help her stand. I am very wary of this one. I remember mid December, when they almost tore her shoulders out of the sockets. I expressed my concerns to the team. They were very cautious. This machine had a remotely operated push button that can be regulated, stopped, and started as needed. They wheeled the contraption in front of her where she was sitting in the chair. With her sling still under her they provide some push as the powered handle bar gives her the assist she needs to stand on her own. The handle bar reminds me of the steering mechanism on a jetski. One of the team stands by in back in case she buckles. She manages to stand and I take a photo at 3:00pm. What a great accomplishment to visualize as I finish my visit for the day. **SHE WAS STANDING!!**

She was shaky, and holding on. When that was completed I was off for the day.

February 11th, I arrived about 11:00am. The counts reported are: Sugar 126, hemoglobin 8.2, and potassium is 3.5.

1:45pm the physical therapy team came by to put her **in a harness machine and walk** while suspended lightly over the floor. I was able to take a brief video of this which I later shared with my wife. She was able to watch her own legs moving ever so slightly across the hallway floor. The "ride" was quite painful. The harness pulled between her legs and groin area. The weight was just enough to give her slight traction. The harness sling took most of the weight. She made it out the door of her room very slowly, and down the hall about 3 feet to a wall supply station. She noted that as her mark of progress. This took about 15 or more minutes. They offered her a wheel chair at that point. She refused, stating she would make the trip back to the room, no matter the pain. What a great pivotal point in her progress. The physical therapy team helped her get into her chair when this was done. This was quite a leap towards the future.

At 2:30 pm she is ready for some Robitussin and a feeding with a bolus product (pouring the liquid food directly down the feed tube).

Speech therapy came by at 3:15pm with the new electric unit and strapped it to her chin. They will conduct 5 separate sessions with this stimulator and then schedule another swallowing test later on, using barium and x-ray. The therapist sat across from her asking her to perform hard swallow efforts. She tried vocal sounds. All through this session the therapist would press a control button to send the electrical stimulus to the throat area.

Sugar count is 162 at 4:40pm.

At 5:07pm the lift team came in to put her back in her bed. Medication was given (Metoprolol, and Carafate). She's had a busy day.

8:45pm sugar count is 171.

At 2:30am the next morning **her heart rate jumped to 177** for a short couple of seconds. The head nurse came in from the station to see if there was some reason. She was worried. No further warnings came. It could have been the machine. This is scary stuff. We are always on guard for some new challenge we don't want.

February 12th the team head doctor came in and said she was pleased with recent progress.

At 9:15am the primary doctor was checking the medical schedule for IVIG and her discharge date. He mentioned a 2nd level hospital locally that would be good for rehab. Our hopes were heightened at the thought of finally getting out of here, but, the health insurance hurdle had to be addressed. The insurance company is showing reluctance to cooperate with the local area rehab centers. We are starting to feel there is a big problem building here.

10:00am medication is a protein shot, Prevacid, folic acid, Carafate, Metoporal, and potassium.

11:15am the speech therapy tech came in to do more swallow therapy with my wife. When that was finished the lift team was there to put her into the chair at 11:45am using the small crane and my wife's sling. It might be good to point out once again, that this "sling" is kept in the room for reuse only by the patient for personal sanitary reasons. Sugar was tested as soon as she got into the chair. It was 157.

I performed some leg therapy on her, moving her legs up and down, while having her push against my efforts. I rotated her ankles and had her "step on the gas", and pull up with her toes against my hand.

I took a lunch break in the hospital cafeteria. At 2:20pm Physical Therapy showed up again with the walking machine they used yesterday. They wanted to take advantage of the availability of the machine. Sometimes these machines are in use by other patients. They try to get them when they can. They liked her progress so much yesterday they want to keep going.. This time they started out allowing more pressure on the legs. It didn't go so well. I suggested they "lift" the adjustment for suspension to take some weight off the legs. I think they were a little to aggressive and looking for improvements from yesterday. The fact is, the muscles are so frail in their rebuilding that they don't rebound so easily 24 hours later

. Three people are involved with the machine this time. One is on his knees in the back being sure all straps are secure and moving correctly. One is operating the electric buttons needed to raise and lower the harness as needed. And the other is supervising and assisting for safety issues from behind. Of course they have to contend with me and my "two cents". After the lift adjustment I suggested, she is able to place one foot in front of the other once again. This time she made the trip down the hall past the wall cabinet she used as a target yesterday. **She kept going to the next doorway and returned**. Wow! It is difficult to convey in writing the chaos and scrambling all the techs put into this procedure to get her to this stage. What a great crew.

I left for the day. She has been doing well and I feel more comfortable.

February 13th I arrived back at the hospital at 10:40am. Hemoglobin is 8.3. I was told the Ear, Nose, and Throat doctor came in last night. He said the vocal cords are shrunken, but there is therapy for that. He said the ears look good.

At 1:15pm blood pressure is 122/57, and temperature is 97.7°. The lift team put her into her chair at 2:00pm. By 5:40pm she was ready to go back to the bed. Sugar tested at 200 and blood pressure is 129/59. The night nurse came in early today at 6:15pm. She gave my wife insulin and antibiotics. The daytime nurse was still on duty and flushed the PEG tube after feeding my wife her bolus dose. 9:50pm, medicine is Prevacid, Metoprolol, insulin, Carafate, and Heparin. A quick bed pan was in order also. She is still not mobile enough to get to the restroom yet. Blood pressure is 117/54, temperature is 98.0°, and sugar reading is 133. We watched a little television and I stayed the night on my sponge covered couch.

.

February 14th the primary doctor arrived early. At 8:10am he says he will check out **an antibiotic to add because of the long duration of steroids**. 9:10am medicine is Prevacid, folic acid, Metoprolol, and Carafate. Blood pressure is 116/52, but she accepted the Metoprolol anyway. By 10:40am blood pressure dropped to 111/51 which is still not too low according to the nurse. Temperature is 98.0°, and heart rate is 70bpm.

I left for the day.

February 15th I arrive at 9:45am to a bed pan session. I waited outside the door until the nurse was finished with her.

The "team" lead doctor came in at 10:00am. She is very pleased with our progress. I told her we might need a letter to our doctors up north explaining the need for her IVIG medication. She will coordinate with case management and provide a letter for our insurance claiming a critical need of IVIG infusions.

My wife told me the Gastro doctor was in last night and is very pleased with the PEG tube placement. He saw **no new signs of infection**.

10:10am blood pressure is 123/53 , heart rate is 89bpm, temperature is 98.0°, hemoglobin is reported at 8.1, potassium 3.5, and sodium 135. Sodium is now the least of our concern. I keep reminding myself it was the low sodium count that brought us in to the hospital in the first place to start this journey. Medications at this time are Metoprolol, Prevacid, folic acid, Prednisone, guafenisen, Carafate, and a bolus feed.

11:25am sugar count is 149. Another bolus feed is given at 1:30pm along with a protein shot. This shot, by the way, is not with a needle. This comes in a small container as a liquid. It is similar looking to the new energy shots so popular at the store check out counters. It is poured into the PEG tube with the bolus feed.

12:00pm the Physical Therapy team showed up with the walking machine again. The main tech is so enthused with my wife and wants to help her anyway she can. We are getting to know her so well. She is very positive in what she is trying to do. This time they are putting **more weight on her legs. I can see them buckle**. One of the techs is trying to tell her to hold the knees in. She is grimacing with the pain, but insists on going on. She started out with her walker inside the walking space. It was in the way. They removed it so they can get involved with the leg movement. She didn't make it as far this time. This was a tough one, but successful none-the-less, given the pressure they put on the legs.

The dietician came by at 1:40pm to discuss feeding. She decided to schedule 6 bolus feedings spaced every 3 hours. That leaves just enough time to get some sleep each night.

It's Monday. That means a chemo shot. The Oncology team came by at 1:50pm to administer the subcutaneous dose of Methotrexate using all the precautions.

2:30pm was a bedpan call.

Speech therapy tech came by at 4:00pm for another stimulus session. Sugar tested at 200 at 4:30pm. They gave her 4 units of insulin at 6:45pm. She also received Prevacid, Nepron, antibiotic, guafenesin, and carafate. At 8:30pm medication is Metoprolol and bolus feed. 10:45pm vitals are 130/57, temperature is 98.4°, and sugar is lower now at 107. The sugar count seems to be lower overnight.

February 16th the morning nurse is reporting hemoglobin at 7.3. I hope it isn't sliding again. This would be another setback we don't want. Sugar this morning is 107. A bedpan is necessary at 10:30am.

The primary doctor reports that **a strong antibiotic, Mepron, is necessary with Methotrexate as a prophylactic protection against outside infections.**

At 11:30am Physical Therapy moved her from the bed to the chair on a slider. I took a brief video of her in the chair **waving her legs and putting them straight out from the sitting**

position. She was actually "waving" her legs playfully out and back. She is definitely getting stronger and in better spirits.

Two people from Speech Therapy came in with the electrode device to keep working on the throat muscles. They taped the electrodes under the chin and encouraged her to swallow while they stimulated the area with the push of a button. They think the progress is there.

12:30pm the nurse is using Heparin to keep the Med-port clear.

When I got home that afternoon, I was able to get a nice wheel-chair from my neighbor. He had bought it for his wife earlier, but upon her recovery he was ready to give it away. What a find. I took a photo of it to show to my wife the next day.

February 17th I arrive at 8:45am. I get the report right away for hemoglobin at 8.2. That's a little better. Sugar is borderline so no shot will be required this time.

8:45am the Speech Therapy tech came in to perform a **vocal cord scope**. She had to set up a monitor and the apparatus. She carefully explained to my wife that she will use a topical numbing solution with a swab. Then she will insert a tube down her throat to examine the throat muscles and vocal chords. All this will be watched on the monitor and recorded on the computer for future evaluation with a doctor. By 9:20am she performed the procedure asking my wife to make various sounds and swallows. **She completed everything in less than ten minutes.**

The primary doctor came in at 9:30am to say **they were considering taking her to the hospital's own rehab facility** since nothing was working out elsewhere. Shortly after he left she was given her bolus feed. I haven't mentioned it for a while, but, respiratory techs showed up 2 or 3 times everyday lately to have her breathe in a mist with medication to avoid pneumonia. It became so often and automatic I failed to put it in my notes each visit.

At 10:10am her blood pressure is 123/54 and temperature is 97.6°. Blood pressure at 2:23pm is

129/51. Those are good numbers. The Physical Therapy team showed up with the walking machine lift at 2:55pm. Once again they attach the sling and raise her to her feet. This time I **notice a lot more strength in her movement** and less pain in her face. She kept her walker in the walking space and used it as if it were her only support. There was a strange sense of normalcy here. She made a much longer stretch down the hallway and back for 20 minutes. I am very proud of her. They worked with her until almost 3:30pm.

It's 4:10pm and the "team" lead doctor stopped in to check on my wife.. She explained the dosage of Methotrexate needed for the future release. She is prescribing 4 x 2.5 mg pills to be taken every Monday. She gave us the letter we asked for and recommended a good doctor to contact back home for follow up when we go back.

4:20 pm sugar count is 182. 4:25pm the nurse fed her the bolus and will ask the doctors about the water intake because the sodium drops when too much "free" water is consumed. The sodium count was 131 today. We worry about that still, but not as much.

5:30pm a head doctor from the **hospital rehab** came in to discuss her future move to his facility. He assured us he has influence in making this happen and she is a good candidate. He told us they have an average patient stay of 3 to 4 weeks. He will be coordinating efforts and **it is likely she will go there**. We are not sure ourselves. There have been so many disappointments.

8:38pm medications are Prevacid, Metoprolol, and Carafate. 9:45pm vitals are blood pressure 118/55, temperature 98.2°, and sugar is 150. 10:30pm medication is Xanax, Heparin, and Robitussin. We watched a little TV together and after some of the news, shut off the TV and went to sleep for the night. I prepared my flip out couch with the sheets and pillows and foam mattress cover they provided me.

February 18th blood pressure at 10:15am is 126/56 and temperature is 98.0°. Hemoglobin is reported at 8.6 and potassium is 3.5. Sugar tested at 150. Things seem to be stabilizing as we approach the possibility of "graduating" to rehab. Medication at this time is Prednisone, Metoprolol, Robitussin, Heparin, and folic acid.

11:00am, the primary doctor reports that **rehab seems to be a "go".** They are waiting for a bed to become ready. The medication continues at that facility just as it would if we were moved to another room within the hospital. He made notes of a comment I made about using vitamin B12 as a way of building the blood count. He wasn't sure that would help. I was passing on a personal story based on the experience of a friend of mine.

12:55pm blood pressure 114/24. It seems low to me. I will watch the next one closely.

I left for home and met my neighbors at our RV park. They had a 4 wheel walker which had a seat and a shopping basket. I took a picture of it to show my wife the next day.

I rolled the walker around in the house. It wouldn't fit through the doorway to the bedroom. I knew **I would have to widen the doorway** because she would need that passage to be independent after she is discharged from rehab. I only needed to cut it open about 2 inches.

February 19th I arrived at the hospital at 8:40am while a team doctor was examining my wife. At 9:10am her blood pressure is 114/59. Although these readings seems low to me, they keep them in that range with the medicine they are giving her. I am used to the readings we both get at the doctor's office during a check-up. They are usually higher.

At 11:00am she was able to get the lift team to put her in the chair. The primary doctor came in 20 minutes later to say the high sugar count is not a problem in a hospital setting. That will be monitored and controlled on the outside as we go forward. With the gradual reduction of steroids, the **sugar counts may become a thing of the past.** At 11:30am her sugar is 153 and hemoglobin is 8.5; not bad.

She left for another swallow study at 1:15pm. We are hoping she can pass this time.

She returned at 1:45pm very excited. She told me she passed the test and could swallow. We are both crying with happiness. She will be starting on ice chips. The head nurse came in to hear the news.

The nurse left the room excited. She returned with a cup of ice chips and my wife took a teaspoon and gently swallowed a couple of chips. I took a picture of the moment.

The Team lead doctor arrived in the room at 2:15pm. She told us we were very close to moving on to rehab in the hospital facility. She had to leave for the week and would probably not see us because we will have moved on by then. She asked my wife if she could have a "hug". She gave me a hug also and turned to say goodbye. As she started to head for the door I sensed tears welling in her eyes. I was very touched by her emotional moment. **This has been a long, difficult journey.**

About 3:00pm the primary doctor came in to tell us she learned of the swallow test. We told her we celebrated with a cup of ice chips. She was quite upset to learn that my wife was consuming ice chips already. She said that although the swallow test was good, she did not want her to swallow anything just yet. She said **if there were any problems of aspiration, it could set everything back**. She preferred caution and guidance from the swallow team and the dietitian as we move forward. I guess we got a little over anxious.

Medications at 4:00pm are folic acid, Carafate and bolus feeding. 4:10pm sugar count is 176. 5:25pm blood pressure is 132/51 and temperature is 97.8°. 6:35pm blood pressure is 125/58. Medication of Tylenol and Benadryl were given to prepare her for the next session of IVIG.. The IVIG was started at 7:30pm. 8:30pm feeding was administered in the PEG tube by the nurse. We actually were getting the IVIG a day early in order to complete the sessions before the transfer to rehab. **That would set the timing for the next session of IVIG to be just before discharge from rehab**. At least that is the plan.

February 20 after a night of sleep on my hospital couch, I folded my blankets and sponge cover. The Nurse brought me a cup of coffee. I got some valuable counts. At 7:30am Hemoglobin is 8.4; potassium is 3.7. Sugar tested at 107; it usually is low in the morning. Medication at 9:14am is Vitamins, Robitussin, Prevacid, Metoprolol, Carafate, and potassium.

It's 11:40am and the lift team came in to put her in the wheel chair. We are going to get out once more for some fresh air. Her brother and his wife are here to visit. They followed us as I pushed her through the hallways and the glow of the moment was contagious as we moved on past the nurse's station and headed for the elevator. She wanted to go to the circular flower garden again. We sat there for a moment and noticed a man and his girlfriend across the way, seated in one of the picnic benches provided here. He was smoking a cigarette, much against the rules. There was a "no-smoking" sign posted right next to him. A nurse sat near us to enjoy her lunch. She overheard me calling his attention to the sign and the policy. He smirked and continued his stubborn abuse of the rules as if to defy the world. The nurse was quite put out by this and put her sandwich down. She said. "That's not going to happen!", and walked to the security station that was not too far away. The security guard came immediately to escort the man and his date off the premises. I thanked her for intervening. I told her my wife just started immunosuppressant therapy and we are concerned for her susceptibility to possible dangers, such as that second hand smoke. We are so new to this we may be overprotective, but, that doesn't dismiss the fact that this man was clearly out of line. We have to be so careful as we learn our limits.

We spent a little time at a bench where we all overlooked the bay on a bright sunny day. We all reminisced about how far she has come.

My brother-in-law and sister stayed to be with her for the IVIG session that afternoon. They gave me a break so I could take care of things at home.

February 21 the day nurse is reporting the hemoglobin at 7.6. The primary doctor came by at 9:30am to saying **everything is steady**. They are not anticipating any delays in going to rehab. It should be any day now as soon as a room becomes available. At 10:50am the blood pressure checks out at 118/51, and temperature is 97.8°. At 2:15pm blood pressure is 108/58. She was supposed to get fed at 2:30pm but they came in late. Sometimes these schedules get pushed around, but her stomach still growls from hunger.

At 3:00pm she received medications, including preparation for the next segment of the IVIG treatment. She got Tylenol, guaifenesin, Carafate, saline solution and Benadryl. She needed a bedpan at 4:10pm and the sugar reading at that time tested at 249.

The IVIG began at 4:15pm. She finally got a feeding at 6:00pm. Vitals taken at 6:20pm after the feeding are blood pressure of 143/57. They weren't too happy with that reading and took another which came out to be 131/59. They like to keep it low.

Most of the time we are occupying now is watching vitals and exercising to build strength in anticipation of getting out of here and into rehab. If rehab's history of stay is 3 weeks, then **we are looking at going home before the end of March.** I find it hard to imagine at this time that she will be strong enough to take care of herself. I am thinking I will be totally involved with her recovery. We still have a long road ahead.

It is 8:30pm and the sugar count is 158, temperature is 98.2°, and blood pressure is 131/56. Medicines given at this time are Prevacid, Metoprolol, Heparin, and Peridex. Peridex is an oral rinse to reduce the amount of bacteria in the mouth.

We watched a little TV together and got some sleep. I am getting used to the couch.

February 22 it's 7:00am and the nurse's are changing-shift. The new day nurse is reporting hemoglobin at 7.8. It seems to be holding. We have a bedpan session at 8:00am. The team doctors came by at 8:30am for their routine checkup. The medicines given at 9:15am are Peridex, Robitussin, potassium, folic acid, Prednisone, vitamins, and Carafate. By now, we know what each of these meds are for. The bedpan was needed again at 9:55am. At 10:00am blood pressure reading is 148/62. Sugar count is

164 at 11:30am, and because it is **Monday she receives her dose of Methotrexate**.

It's 1:30pm and the team lead doctor's replacement came in for a check up. This was the first visit for this doctor. The check up was very thorough. It seems we are getting closer to "graduation". The check ups indicate a much stronger patient. I still feel I would be at a disadvantage if I had to take her home at this moment, however. I hope she can get to a better level. The mystery is: **what will that level be?.**

After the doctor left it was time for another bedpan session. A few minutes later the blood pressure checks out at 131/52, and the temperature is 98.3°.

It's 2:30pm and I decided to give her legs a thorough PT session before I leave for the day. I left at 2:45pm. I actually have the possibility of playing a game of golf tomorrow with some of my friends. That will be a change.

Chapter Eight

REHAB

It is February 23 and I am checking the home hallway width for the 4 wheel walker. I definitely will have to modify the passageway to the bedroom. We are anticipating moving her to rehab any day, so I have to be ready.

I arrived at the golf course about 1:00pm to await my T-time. A short while later I got a wonderful text from my wife. **She is moving to rehab today**. Finally, we are on our way. I announced the good news to all my golfing friends. The golf game went well.

February 24th, after showering and getting ready to go back to the hospital, I took pictures of the 4 wheel walker at the doorway. I plan on showing them to my wife. I arrived at the hospital about 10:30am to find her in her new room at the hospital rehab center. On the "white-board" is a schedule of rehab training that consists of 5 separate 45 minute sessions including physical therapy, occupational therapy, and speech therapy.

At 11:00am they moved her to a wheel chair with the assistance of a canvas belt wrapped around her waist. She had to put pressure on her legs, no more lift team. At 11:15am two doctors came in to give her a thorough examination and evaluation to be used in gauging her progress while in this unit.

1:45pm she is taken to the gym. We make sure she has her mask on and surgical gloves for her own protection while being exposed to all the people and equipment, and any contamination she might encounter. We are cautious of her immune condition. Although they wipe everything down with disinfecting wipes, we aren't taking any chances. Fifteen minutes later her nurse came into the gym with her feed from upstairs. Since she is still on PEG feeding, the nurse merely opened the dose of food and poured it into the funnel which attaches to the feed tube going into her stomach. She placed the binder back over the tube and my wife was able to continue therapy which is designed to strengthen her legs. I took a picture of her pumping her legs on the bicycle pedal machine. The therapy schedule is very disciplined. If the food is late, they bring it to where ever the patient is doing exercises.

2:40pm is speech therapy. Then at 3:00pm doctors came in to review their plans. Then speech therapy continues after the doctors leave. Speech therapy will continue for now with ice chips. Then they will evaluate swallows again to eliminate retention problems. It is good to have the rehab facility as part of the hospital environment. Some of the same people who are familiar with her case will be in attendance as she progresses, especially speech therapy.

8:45pm it is time for medication of Heparin, Carafate, Prevacid, and B12. I have an open bed in the room, so I can sleep over. Once again a good break for me, given the distance I have to travel everyday. I can cut my commute burden in half by spending every other night here.

February 25, 7:45am I met the morning duty nurse. She told me the hemoglobin count is 7.8. I am still on the alert for this one, even if we have graduated to rehab. The schedule is on the wall again. They have a serious regimen. I brought my laptop to catch up on my work. I use the time that she is occupied, to get bills paid, catch up on e-mail, etc. When she is taken to various parts of the building I go with her. When the therapy routine is scheduled in the room, I keep myself busy and out of their way.

At 7:50am Occupational therapy came in to help her dress and lift her to the wheel chair. She is very weak but showing signs of being able to help the move using her new muscles as much as she can. The legs are the weakest.

Physical therapy came to the room at 8:30am to take her to the gym. They wheeled her chair to the parallel stand rails. There is enough room between the rails for the wheel chair to fit. The therapist wiped down the rails with disinfectant before she touched them. She is not wearing latex gloves for protection. She is wearing a surgical mask. The therapist helps her stand by facing her inside the rails. He places his gloved hands under her arms above her waist with his fingertips gently under the canvas belt around her ribs. It is just above the stomach binder which she is constantly wearing to protect the PEG tube in her stomach.

He helps her to her feet. With his help she is able to maintain a somewhat shaky standing position while holding her weight up with her hands on the rails. My attention is brought to the bare hands, and I mention it to the therapist. He apologetically admits the error. **He offers her some antiseptic foam to wash on her hands, and gets her a pair of gloves** from the box nearby. After a little over a half hour of various other exercises such as squeezing balls and catching and throwing, we returned to the room.

9:30am medication is vitamins, Carafate, potassium, and Prevacid. All of these are in the records followed by computer from the main hospital. This is a good advantage to continuing her therapy in the attached hospital facility. After assisting in a potty call at 10:10am I am ready to head for home. I have to buy some plywood on the way home to start building a ramp for the wheelchair. Before I leave **I made sure to organize the many sheets and blankets, plus other supplies scattered around the room**. The last one in the room casually set aside this stuff somewhere. It seems these nurses and aids are always searching for towels, wipes, and the like. It is no different here than it was in the main hospital when it comes to organization. .

When that is done I gathered my computer, briefcase, lunch cooler, and her laundry, and with a kiss on her cheek, I leave for home.

Now that she is rehabilitating, I am required to provide clean street clothes for her. Of course, with the loss of weight, nothing really fits. **I will have to buy some new clothes for her.**

February 26th my wife called me by phone, in the morning, to tell me her hemoglobin number went back up. It is 8.1 this morning. She knows what to look for by now. She said she went to the gym with Physical Therapy and **walked 6 steps** using a walker. The therapist followed closely behind with a wheelchair. The idea was to give moral support and an emergency seat if she lost strength or balance. It sounds like great progress.

In the meantime I was busy at our house sawing plywood. I had to make a portable ramp in the front door. The two steps are a short distance from the door, so I had to cut a handle in the surface of the ramp for my hand. I can lift the ramp away more easily when not in use, and then the door can close. Our place is rather small quarters. This will have to do for now. We won't be here long. We will have to get to our northern home soon to get "in-network" attention since the insurance carrier has its limitations on care here.

Our concern now is for the follow up outpatient rehab we will require in our home town environment.

I took some pictures of the ramp to show my wife when I get to her room tonight.

I arrived at her room around 5:30pm after my

long day of constructing the ramp. It's a long walk from the parking lot to the rehab center. I will have to check out the shuttle car next trip, especially when I am carrying extra supplies. We shared some of the stories of the day. I showed her the pictures of the ramp. She filled me in on her routines of the day.

8:30pm is medicine time. She gets Heparin, Carafate, and Prevacid. We then watched a little TV. I made my bed up for the night. Our room shares a midway bathroom. When I use the bathroom I have to lock the other patient's door, and when I am done, I must unlock that door so they can use the room when they need to. When they do use the bathroom they will have to do the same routine locking the door to my wife's room. Cleanliness is not at the same level as it was in the main hospital. I feel much more on guard to wash everything I touch, and wash my hands when I touch anything. I am consciously keeping my hands away from my face, and I wear gloves as much as I can so as not to contaminate my wife. She has enough problems to work on. This environment is more like a gymnasium locker room.

The morning of February 27th the doctor reports hemoglobin at 7.3. He will order a midday blood sample to test it again to establish a pattern. He also reports that a random test they did showed her positive for C-diff infection. I learned this is one of the worst offenders a person can get in the hospital. It is a bacterium called *Clostridium difficile* (*C. difficile*, or *C. diff*). Though relatively rare compared to other intestinal bacteria, C-diff is one of the worst causes of infectious diarrhea in the U.S. He asks her many questions about stomach cramps, diarrhea, dehydration, etc. **She is showing no outward signs** of such problems. However, we are now instructed to wear a protective gown whenever in her presence. They have also changed the supply of gloves to a thicker type to avoid any chance that a tear could jeopardize anyone's health. Until this time, I avoided wearing the gowns when sitting off in the chair with my computer and magazines. The nurses and aides were constantly wearing them, since the environment is their constant challenge. I, on the other hand, only stay with my wife. They are attending to others in the hospital, so they have to guard against transmission of these germs. Now, they are insisting that I cover always for the sake of protecting everyone involved. These gowns cause a person to sweat if you're not moving around with some air passing through. So, obviously, I had to move around after sitting with a hot laptop for any length of time. I didn't like this situation, but I am not the sick one here.

11:00am Occupational training came by for about a half hour. They were followed very closely by Physical Therapy. PT had to be performed in the room because of the fear of spreading the C-diff infection. He walked her back and forth in the room and performed other strengthening exercises which he told her she could continue on her own during the after hours to help the progress of rehabilitating her muscles.

At 3:45pm we are told the latest hemoglobin reading is 9.5. This second test only makes us think that the hemoglobin is fluctuating each day depending on her activity. We are getting less concerned over this number. (Perhaps the previous doctor was right when he shared his thoughts. He concluded that her bone marrow's ability to replace blood [hemoglobin] might be weaker than most people). She also tends to get a little more rest here.

It is now time for me to go home.

I left straight for the department store. My wife wanted some exercise pants and a secure pair of new sneakers to give her more support as she progresses in standing and walking. Upon arriving home I took pictures of the new items and sent them to her cellphone. About an hour later she sent me a text to ask for pictures of her closet so she can tell me what clothing she would like for her room. She instructed me on the ones to pick. I laid them on the bed and took a picture of them and sent it for her approval. It must be a good feeling for her to be planning a future. It didn't appear that way to her a couple of months ago.

February 28 I left for the Hospital Rehab. It is about an hour drive. I can do this one with my eyes closed. (I wouldn't recommend it!). I took the selected clothing with me. She was pleased to have her own wardrobe. She had a bag of laundry waiting for me. I now had a new duty of bringing fresh things for her to wear each day.

We spent part of the day chatting between rehab sessions. We had to start planning for her return to the house. We weren't sure what the capacity will be. She had been talking with her sister about needs. Her sister had a chair for use in the tub. It would allow my wife to sit from the outside and swing into the tub to take her shower. The tub had sliding glass doors, which meant they would have to be replaced with a plastic curtain for flexibility. Her sister also had a bed rail to be inserted between the mattress and box spring. That secures it so the rail portion angles upward, and the feet of it touch the floor for stability. The patient can use it for support upon entering or leaving the bed. These were left from her husband who passed away a couple of years ago. Equipment did not seem to be as hard to come by as I had previously thought.

Her sister came by to visit later that afternoon. She brought the bed rail and the tub chair. After a visit of about an hour, she was ready to leave. I planned my exit accordingly. We left together and met at the entrance. I pulled my car up next to her car and took the items. I thanked her and left for home with the new equipment.

After stopping for some things on the way, I arrived at the house. I took the items in. The bed rail was easy to install. It was almost 9:00pm when I sent the pictures of the new equipment to my wife to give her a sense of the progress we are making, and give her a feeling of healing.

February 29 I took the day off from the hospital visit. I had to catch up on finalizing the fit of the wheelchair ramp plus other chores to make things ready as the timing that was appearing to develop for her eventual return home got closer. It seems like things are moving much faster now, or it could be the pressure closing in on me.

She called me to say she wrenched her back. It is very painful to try to turn either way.

March 1st and I am back at the hospital. It's

mid-afternoon and the nurse is reporting hemoglobin at 7.6. My wife is finished with her rehab schedule and ready for a somewhat relaxing evening with me. Her back is still very tender. I suggested she may have cracked a bone. Steroids make the bones brittle. At 4:26pm she is given Carafate. Her sodium is checking out at 137, right on target. At 5:55pm she is being given Nepron, Metoprolol, and being fed through the PEG tube. One thing we are concerned with is the sugar content. The nurse is using Gatorade to rinse the PEG tube and prevent clogging. However we need something sugar free. I suggested PowerAde Zero. They don't have that in the kitchen. **Imagine a hospital not able to cope with this diabetes' balance. I will have to buy it myself.** This will be my ongoing assignment while she is here. You would think they would have a sugar free item in the kitchen, given the concerns for proper food intake. This is very puzzling.

It is 9:25pm and she is getting insulin and Heparin.

March 2nd 1:30am she is up for a bedpan

session. 5:30am, and it is a medication and a bedpan session. She is looking forward to getting strong enough to use the potty. Her sugar count this morning is 86. It is 7:00am and the day nurse says they have scheduled an MRI to look at her back. Apparently my comment did not go unanswered. 7:15am, they are taking her for the MRI.

She's back. The procedure was over in about a half an hour. At 8:36am a neurology doctor stopped in to check on her. At 9:15am the hemoglobin report is 7.5. It is still low but it has been stable. The medication at this time is folic acid, vitamins, Heparin, and potassium.

March 3rd the doctors are reporting no damage seen in the MRI, or the X-rays they took yesterday. They have concluded that this was a muscle strain and it should subside. The rehab training will take this into consideration during exercises. They took her for an ultra sound to examine the area of pain. I am pleased with their concern.

March 4th the day nurse is reporting sugar count at 89, hemoglobin holding nicely at 7.8, and blood pressure is 134/62. She is getting her food through the PEG tube, and her medication is Levimere, and multivitamins.

The doctor of internal medicine was in to say C-diff is not showing symptoms. They will complete treatment of 14 days on Flagyl (this is the medicine used to combat C-diff), and continue cleansing disciplines with hot water and soap, Clorox does not work as well with this bacteria. The primary doctor is cutting the pain medication. He also reports that the ultra sound taken yesterday shows bruising in her back, so, he says it will heal.

March 5th I arrive at 1:00pm. The nurse tells me the hemoglobin count is 7.6. My wife and I chat between therapy sessions. Although I don't note it every day, these sessions are at least 5 total. They are of various disciplines, and last 30-45 minutes each. All the technicians are very serious about giving the total time and input for maximum results. The timing between sessions can be as little as 15 minutes, or as much as 45 minutes.

They feed her through the PEG tube at 5:10pm. Her blood pressure is 114/51 BP. At 10:15pm her medications are:. Prevacid, Carafate, Flagyl, and insulin,

I stayed the night.

March 6th, we are up and at it early. She is using all the tools they have given her to get dressed. She has a grocery pincher to help pick her clothing items up. This is the old fashioned item we are all familiar with that has a trigger type handle with a long reach to a hinged spring action clip at the far end to snag the items. She also has a half cylinder on a rope which is used to put on her socks. The half cylinder goes into the sock. With the rope handle in her hand, she drops the "loaded" cylinder near the floor and carefully inserts her foot into the sock as she pulls back on the rope, which removes the half cylinder leaving the sock on the foot. It is like a large "shoe-horn" on a string.

8:30am the doctors came by to clear her for the gym. Until now they feared the results of the C-diff test, but she had shown no signs of distress. They have concluded that since this bacteria exists within many of us, the body keeps it in check with its own bacteria. They thought she would have more trouble with her immune system being down. **Maybe this is a sign of how strong she really is getting.**

At 9:30am it is time for medication. She gets Lovenox (blood thinner instead of Heparin), Carafate, Flagyl, long acting insulin, and a feeding through the PEG tube. Physical therapy is scheduled for 11:00am.

I left for home about 1:00pm.

Monday, March 7th. , I arrived at 12:45pm. The nurse tells me the Hemoglobin count is 8.5. This is getting more reliable all the time. She is getting Methotrexate today. Lunch feeding is through the PEG tube. She walked the perimeter of the gym earlier today using her walker and techs on all sides.

3:45pm, the **Infectious Disease** doctor stopped

in. He said he doesn't know why they tested for C-diff. Some people have it but so minor they don't show symptoms. The tests are so sensitive, they show the smallest amount. The random check had brought some **unnecessary fears**. Many people's systems are able to keep it in check.

March 8th. 7:00am, we are up and ready for another day of workouts. 8:15am physical therapy made her stand-up 10 times from a sitting position. At 8:30am the **internal medicine doctor** says they will hold off on blood thinners one more day. He said: "The C-diff was a 'false?' reading. It is present but not active. Many of us carry it in our system". It was such a scary thing for us to come across. This had me researching on-line, talking to friends and relatives, and getting feedback from many sources. The information wasn't "pretty". I'm glad she is "off the hook". They all seemed quite concerned.

9:00am medications are: Folic acid, long term insulin, Prevacid, potassium, Prednisone, and Carafate. After her "lunch" (via PEG tube) they came by at 1:00pm to take her to the gym for physical therapy all decked out in her protective gown. Although she was cleared on the C-diff results, they had not taken the gown and gloves requirement off the computer yet, so we were stuck with this directive: gown, protective gloves, and facemask.

She was guided on a walk around the gym. One tech had a hold on her canvas waist belt while she walked on her own using a walker. Another tech followed her nearby with the wheel chair, ready to slip it under her if she weakened. She looked remarkably mobile.

After spending the time to observe her progress in the gym, I gave her a thumb's up and a wave. I left for home.

The rest of the next few days is very much a repeat each day. She followed a routine feeding and medicine schedule, along with 4 to 5 sessions of various types of therapy, improving a little more each day.

March 11th was highlighted by a major swallow study at 1:00pm. She was taken to a room with a **live x-ray screen** that will be on during the physical swallow test. She received a barium enriched pudding which she was to swallow with instructions over a loud speaker while the technician stayed behind in another room. A doctor observed the progress on the television monitor in that room. I was privileged to be there to witness this. I took a video of the progress as we watched the substance being prepared in her mouth. The tech told her to swallow when she was ready. We watched it move to the back of the mouth and down the throat as a muscle in the throat pushed out and squeezed it down the esophagus. This took her about 30 seconds. What a great feeling to see this, another hurdle accomplished. It was an amazing piece of science to be privileged to observe. **She received the final "green light" to advance to solid foods. What a thrill.**

Later that afternoon we received a visit from the dietician to explain the types of food she will try.

March 12th, 7:30am, **breakfast is served**. Here we go. They bring in a tray consisting of whipped foods. There was a side dish of applesauce, a cup of coffee, a cup of ice chips, and a pre-sealed cup of pudding. For the main course: sausage and eggs. Not the way we think of it. Each item was like a molded pudding. The egg was yellow and fluffy. It was about 2 or 3 inches across and about ½" thick. The sausage was also whipped and seemed to be placed out of a mold onto the plate. It had the physical appearance of sausage links lined up side by side. There was to be no chances taken for food not thoroughly chewed before swallowing. This was to be the first taste of "real" food. The Speech therapist attended this HISTORIC event. My wife carefully placed a small amount of egg in her mouth. She said it was bland. She then tried the sausage. You would have to be there to appreciate the look on her face. It was not complimentary. She never liked sausage anyway. It is a good thing they included a couple of containers of "Boost" for her to drink. The food situation was going to be a learning proposition after not eating for almost 4 months.

Nothing "tasted" good to her. The plate presentation was so interesting I had to take a picture of it.

March 15th we attended a committee meeting at 10:00am. These committee meetings are very regimented and allow little time for questions. They do all the talking. It is designed to keep us informed. They try to make the rounds to every patient in the facility in that morning. The primary doctor .told us the **discharge is scheduled for Friday, March 18th.** We were still trying get our future established for outside rehab which she definitely needs.

I had heard from a nurse that there was another woman on the same floor with my wife's affliction. I asked if she could arrange a meeting with her. I would certainly want to compare some stories and get an inside look at what she went through. The nurse said she would check it out, but cautioned me that they protect the privacy of the patient and would only allow it if the patient agreed.

A few more days of rehab routines and her strength is growing. We were looking forward to Friday.

March 16th, 9:45am, Wednesday, the nurses came in to give her a "Graduation Certificate" from the "In-Patient Rehabilitation Program". She proudly held it up in front of her so I could to take a picture. **We are close to going home**.

Just before lunch the primary doctor came in to review some of her vitals and congratulate her on the pending discharge. We took a moment to explain to him the need for a discharge time of noon. We had a welcome home party waiting for us that afternoon at the clubhouse in our complex.

I asked the nurse about that other patient in rehab with Necrotizing Myopathy. She told me the patient had a relapse and had to return to the main hospital for further care.

I am now thinking my wife is going to be one of the lucky ones.

March 17th , Thursday was a highlight of her stay. At 10:00am the nurses presented her with a "Grad" T-shirt. The sign printed on the front said "**G**o for it, **R**each it, **A**chieve it, **D**emonstrate it". These were stacked vertically so the first letter of each statement, when read from top to bottom, read: G R A D. She happily posed for another picture.

On the wall the crayon-board had the days schedule written: 8:00 OT, 9:00 PT, 10:30 PT, and 11:15 ST. There was no letting up on the last day!

Speech therapy came by just before lunch to assist her eating. The tech taped the stimulator under her chin to help the swallowing muscles. The PEG tube was still available for the supplemental food, and medicines, as needed.

March 18th, Friday, **it is Graduation day**. Naturally things take a long time to get done. There was a lot of paperwork. We received a discharge book with all the medications spelled out. It also included a collection of prescriptions to cover the medicines we will need. There were also plenty of things to carry out of there. We needed to get out in time to make the welcome home party. The discharge was about an hour later than we hoped for. Although we had a built in cushion of time anticipating this sort of thing, it still used up that and more. We called ahead and the group waited for us to get there. They had a warm reception planned. Everyone greeted her. There were many tearful moments of joy.

Chapter Nine

MAKING PROGRESS AS AN OUTPATIENT

March 18th, Friday, it is Graduation day. We got out a little later than we allowed to get to the party as planned. They waited for us and had a warm reception planned. Everyone greeted her. There were many tearful moments of joy. The park residence had been following her story closely. Those that had visited her kept the rest informed. The welcome home group collected some money for us and mounted it on a small tree. What a nice gesture. My wife wore her mask. We weren't taking any chances. People tried to hug her, but I asked for her space. We are unsure of her immune system at this point.

Someone mentioned a power scooter was available in the complex. They quoted me a price of $250.00. I hesitated because she was making such great progress. I was thinking the scooter might be a waste of time, because we will be leaving for our northern home soon. If she continues to progress, the scooter would be an unnecessary investment.

Later that day someone came to us to say the owner of the scooter would let us have it for the cost of the batteries they just put in it. We spent $100 and purchased the scooter. It was reasonable, and a more sensible investment at that price.

We spent the next few days getting oriented in the house. I had to **pull** her up, backwards on my home made ramp to get into our small dwelling. The ramp was rather steep in these small quarters. I installed non-slip pads on the surface to get a better grip with my shoes. We will be leaving in about two weeks. We will have to deal with this for now.

I had to type a list of medicines, dosage, and timing. We received a list of medicines and instructions from the rehab center. This was pages long. **I needed all this on a check list** on the kitchen counter so I could give her everything on schedule.

She had to learn to move around using her walker. One of the walkers was more advantageous outside for shopping. It had 4 wheels, a shopping basket across the front rail, and hand brakes for safety. It seems when we went out this would be easy to use. It was also easily collapsible.

Even though we brought the walker with us to the shopping centers, there were powered shopping units available in the major stores. This became a more convenient option.

March 19th was a busy day for us. Her brother set up **a golf tournament to raise money** to help offset some of her medical expenses. We arrived that morning using her wheel chair.

Many people came to the benefit tournament especially to see my wife. Many made the trip from some distance.

She was careful to wear a face mask, and protective latex gloves avoiding any opportunity for infection. I hovered over her with great care, stopping anyone from hugging or touching her.

She is still frail and subject to infection until she can build up her immunity. I may be over protective, but caution will outweigh some future illness from this exposure.

After the players came in from the tournament, we had a dinner in the reception room. I read a short written speech to the audience to say what I wanted in as few words as possible. It helped control my emotions of the moment. I thanked all who attended. I thanked all who prayed for her everyday. Many of them I had updated, through cellphone texting, on a daily basis previously. I turned to my wife and held the microphone for her to say something. Just before she spoke, I interrupted and I asked her if she wanted to try to stand to do this. She agreed. I held the canvas belt that she still wore for stability when these moments happened. **As she struggled and rose to her feet, you could hear the gasps in the audience**. I even heard someone exclaim, "She's standing!" They were focused. My wife thanked them all for their prayers and visiting. She received a very warm round of applause.

There was karaoke provided for the remainder

of the reception. I sang "Believe" by Brooks and Dunn. There were no dry eyes, including my own.

March 20th we heard there were some guys putting on a "Jam Session" down the street in our RV Park. We got the new scooter out and she rode it to the scene. Many were pleased and excited to see her come. They moved their chairs around and made room for her to back in. I was asked to get up and sing. I sang "I can't stop loving you". She was thrilled.

For the next few days it was necessary to make plans to return to our In-Network area where our insurance could support us through out-patient therapy. We were blessed with very caring friends. One couple offered to drive our car, and anything we would pack in it, 1200 miles back to our northern home. They would fly back at their own expense. Another couple said they would take us to the airport. Her brother bought our airplane tickets. The plans were set.

March 26th was Easter Eve. Her foot was

starting to swell. I feared the worse. I thought she might be regressing. We went to the hospital. Her brother and his wife met us there. We were all concerned. Despite our summary of her illness, the nurses and doctors pursued a more obvious cause. With a sonogram they discovered a blood clot in the upper calf, just behind the right knee. We learned that the IVIG has tremendous clotting properties, and **the rehab center had sent her home without any regard to blood thinner maintenance.** They admitted her and wanted to know if we had a primary doctor to contact. We asked for the doctor that began with us when we entered this regional hospital last November. He was on duty this weekend.

She spent the night in the hospital with shots of blood thinners and a 24 hour observation period. I had to leave at 9:45pm to get her medicines from home. The hospital didn't have the antibiotic she was taking. I brought back some bolus feed for her since it was way past the hospital dinner time and they were not prepared to feed her at that time of night. I fed her through the PEG tube. We were attended by the primary doctor that started with her journey. He worked with us to get us out on Easter morning with a supply of blood thinners. He set us up with prescriptions for Coumadin blood thinner. He asked us about the original diagnosis he and his colleagues guessed at last November. He wanted to know how close they were to the correct answer. He was pleased to hear they were on the right track.

I went home at 10:45pm and returned the next morning, March 27th, at 9:00am. She felt bloated. They had added too much water into the feed tube. I helped her to the bathroom and we waited for our final instructions. After some discharge paperwork we left the hospital at Noon.

We were able to make our date for Easter dinner at her brother's place.

For the next few days before leaving for our northern home, we had to take daily blood tests, since being discharged on **Coumadin blood thinner**. We contacted the primary doctor we had set up down south and he followed our progress.

He telephoned us and recommended the dosage we needed, based on the blood test results he received daily. He needed an address of our primary doctor in the north in order to follow the treatment when we got home. We had to go with the one that she was using when she got in this trouble. It was necessary, in order to make the transition. We were not going to make it permanent. We would look for a new primary doctor when we got there.

On the second night we did have a moment when **a cut on her leg would not stop bleeding**. We wrapped it tight and I recommended she not take a Coumadin pill that night.

The next morning there was **some blood in the bed**. It had not stopped bleeding right away, but was stable when we woke up. This was a scary moment. The doctor called early that morning and said according to the results of the last blood test he recommends cutting the dosage in half. We told him the situation and that we already did that. He was glad. We were in control now and ready to leave for the north. We used our common sense to ward off this major situation.

Wednesday March 30, our very good friends arrived at our southern home according to plan. We got to the Airport early, with almost three hours to spare. Besides the clothes on our backs, she had an overnight bag and I had all the meds. We had arranged for special attention for the handicapped. I had the meds in a small duffle bag, and all the paperwork to back them, in a dedicated brief case. The "shake down" took almost 2 hours. She was patted down in a separate area. They asked her to stand-up from the wheelchair so they could pat her down. I was placed in a circle painted on the floor and asked to remain still while they patted me down. In the meanwhile another guard was going through my duffle bag of nearly $2000 worth of necessary medicines. Despite the length of time, it went smoothly. It just required time and patience, and I was nervous.

.

When we got through, and we were at the inside of the airport, I wanted to stop and get a beer to relax. We didn't have much time left.

One beer would do. Just then, one of the golf tournament visitors spotted us. She came over to say hello. What a break. I asked her if she would escort my wife to the ladies room. I didn't know how I was going to pull that off otherwise. We were able to board the plane comfortably.

Her sister picked us up at our home airport in the north. The airlines had checked our private wheelchair and had it in the tunnel when we came out of the plane. We stopped for lunch on the way home. (There were no groceries at home yet.) My wife ate one of her favorites: "Loaded Potato Soup". It was soft, liquid, and palatable for her condition. When we arrived at our house our sister-in-law's spare car was sitting in the driveway for our needs. We could comfortably wait for our friends to arrive from the south with our car. Our niece and her friends had also cleaned our house for our comfort prior to our arrival. So many people came forward to help us; we are overwhelmed with gratitude.

We had called ahead weeks ago to set up doctors and PT as soon as we got back. Now is the time to review the schedule and set plans. We set up a calendar for the appointments ahead. We devoted one shelf in our kitchen cupboard to hold the medicines. The morning meds were on the left, and the night meds on the right. Each bottle is marked to reflect the dosage and when to take the pill. I used red marker to indicate morning and a black marker for night. There was one med taken 3 times a day, so I put a dose indication in "blue" marker. I put the printed "spreadsheet" in the cupboard with the medicine. I would take this sheet out at medicine time and put it on the counter while I set up the required timely dosage, using the sheet as a sort of map. The dosages were put into the traditional pill dispensers. I used one color dispenser for morning and another for night. I then designated the time I needed to administer the medication.

Along with the medication I included the bolus feed. Some pills needed to be crushed. This was tricky. I put the pills in a "Ziploc" bag and gently hit them with a hammer. The cracked pills, turned gradually to powder. The "Ziploc" bag didn't put up much of a fight. The sharp pieces of the pills poked at the bag. The powder had to be moved around as I hit it. The bag lasted 2 or 3 times before I had to resort to a new one. I was on my own now. I had to administer the meds like the nurses had done for the last few months. I had to be sure to rinse the tube out carefully when I was finished. My wife would hold the PEG tube while I managed the medicine into the opening. We were nervous, but a good team.

April 3rd I have a picture of my wife already cooking spaghetti in the kitchen. She is standing inside her walker while she is stirring the pot. She couldn't wait to start cooking when she got better. She spent many a day in the hospital watching cooking shows on TV and writing recipes down when she could.

April 6th was the first day of local out patient physical therapy at 10:00am. We found the local hospital had an adequate facility. Our insurance carrier was compatible. We paid the required co-pay and we were good to go. They evaluated her muscle tone and gave her some exercises to do.

The exercises were targeted at specific muscle areas. She learned the movements there and got instructions to continue these at home. We also met with the speech therapist there. She determined that my wife was doing well enough to continue throat exercises from a sheet of instructions. We can do this at home and save some separate co-pay money. We scheduled our next PT meeting before leaving for home.

April 7th was our meeting with the new neurologist in our northern city. He is the **best of the best**. We lucked out. We were on our way to continued care. He evaluated her muscle tone just as the other ones had done before, on a scale of 1 to 5. He also boosted her Methotrexate to 15mg, and cut her steroid dose of 40mg to 30mg for one week, then we were to drop it down to 20mg until the next visit in June. **He also put a stop to further IVIG treatment. He sighted the blood clotting problem** and said it would be too dangerous anymore. We set up an appointment for 8 weeks away on June 9.

We had to do some clever shopping. We were

looking for the best prices on "Boost" formula. That was the brand recommended at the hospital for her bolus feeding. We compared labels of other brands. There were alternatives but they didn't taste good. We used them for the bolus feed until they were used up. At this point we were doing mostly meds through the PEG tube. She was trying to "eat" by mouth. We have a blender I used to whip every food item into a drink form. She took the Boost product with her to supplement her food intake, which often wasn't adequate when away from home.

April 11th we saw the original primary doctor. We made some medicine adjustments. There was an antibiotic that cost over $1000 a month that we eliminated. He saw it as preventative, which is not the purpose of an antibiotic. (Although the original purpose the hospital prescribed it for was to hold off any opportunistic infections, given her weakened immune system, and prolonged use of steroids). We got her scripts renewed. He also prescribed Xarelto as a better alternative to Coumadin.

On April 13th I drove her to a local pub where her ladies' golf league was having their planning meeting. She walked in with her walker. She surprised everyone. They had all heard of her problem and were so happy to see her. They discussed keeping her in the league. Someone would substitute for her in the beginning until she was strong enough to play. That was comforting and an incentive to get well. Some of these same women go on an organized golf trip in July for a weekend away. My wife has been attending this for years. With the uncertainty of the future they invited her to this year's trip. All of this was so positive for her. She has a lot of strengthening to do if she is to go. There is so much unknown. No one has been able to give us a firm assessment of the future.

April 15th I have a picture of her eating a fish fry dinner. She was getting much more confident in her swallowing ability. We are getting close to wanting the PEG tube removed. The fish was soft. She took great care to mash or chew each item.

She said she didn't feel nervous about it. This is progress.

April 18th; is more Out Patient PT consisting of leg exercises and instructions for homework.

April 25th we went shopping for a new easy chair for her. **She was pulling her back muscles attempting to raise the foot rest on her old chair**. This might be easy enough for the average person, but her body has a fraction of the muscle mass. We found an **electric style easy chair** at a reasonable price. All she has to do is hold a button to raise her feet. This will save her back.

April 26th: Out Patient PT.

April 29th: Out Patient PT.

May 2nd;is more Out Patient PT followed by an

appointment **with a new primary doctor**. The location is coincidentally across the street from the physical therapy address. This doctor is very thorough. We had heard good reports of this doctor from discussions with other satisfied patients. We were satisfied that we found the right one. We made arrangements to request my wife's records from the original primary doctor.

We were told by the original doctor's secretary that the preparation of the paperwork could take several weeks. This was a problem we had to accept and work with. The move was absolutely necessary in our opinion.

May 4th, we went to see a doctor to get the PEG tube removed. We obtained the reference from our new primary doctor. The visit was rather simple, given the anticipation we both had. Once the required paperwork was complete we went into the patient room and waited for the doctor. Instead, a physician's assistant came in with a trainee. This was a little unnerving. My wife lay on the patient table. The PA pulled my wife's blouse up to examine the area and explain the procedure to her trainee and us. The trainee then tried to pull the tube out giving it a firm tug. It wouldn't budge. He was a little timid, and lacked the experience. My wife's face wrinkled up with the anticipation of pain. Although there was some sensation in the area, she said it didn't hurt much. With some concern for results, the PA decided to do it herself. As the assistant watched, the PA took a good grip on the tube and **popped the PEG tube out** with a long, firm pull. We were surprised it was so simple. It just required a stronger tug. We asked about leakage or infection dangers because of our past experience. These were obvious questions they expect from the patient. We were told **the hole closes up within a few days, by its self**. After a couple of days of precaution in the shower, we will have nothing to fear. This all seemed so mechanical. It was almost like they had drilled a hole in a car's gas tank to get the fuel in while they worked on the regular gas cap. Now the repair was done so the new hole gets plugged and everything is operational again. The weird feeling is: this is a human body. **It shouldn't be that simple**. But there we were back to normal again. They applied a gauze dressing to the area and sent us on our way. What a great feeling to get rid of that thing. **My wife felt like a normal human being again.** She smiled all the way home.

May 5th: more Out Patient PT.

Weather-wise May 9th was a pleasant day at our northern home. **I caught her outside swinging a golf club.** I laughed and took a picture of this milestone. **One of her biggest incentives for getting better was to be able to play golf again**. She never had a powerful swing, but it was accurate. From what I observed, this was true to her old form. Now we would have to see if she had the stamina to play a full game. This was also the first day she got behind the wheel and took the car to the store on her own. It wasn't far, but it was a start.

May 10th: more Out Patient PT.

May 11th she went out to the camper to test

the stairs. I didn't know it until she came in the house to tell me she had negotiated the stairs successfully. She was anxious to know she could go camping again when we are ready.

May 16th: **the LAST Out Patient PT.** The therapists were in agreement. My wife had reached a point where normal daily living and personal exercise will be adequate.

May 27th we attended our niece's wedding and reception. She did not wear a protective face mask this time. **She danced the electric slide.** . I took a video of it. She looked great. She had to wear a new wig, because the chemo had thinned her hair greatly. We were still in agreement she had to be on guard not to allow too many hugs or kisses. There were many friends and relatives there who hadn't seen her yet since hearing of her ordeal.

June 2nd we made an appearance at a local

beach bar with plenty of outside air. This was a fund raising event our niece organized to pay for a children's play set for the local park. One of our favorite bands headed up the venue. It is a very public place. We still have to be on guard. There were a lot of local acquaintances we hadn't seen yet. We avoided any close facial contact. A quick hug was about the most she accepted. **This was a good break in our new medical routine.**

June 8th we took a small tour boat cruise up and down our local riverfront. They had a good band and we were with many of our close friends who followed her plight. **This was a very crowded environment.** So far our cautions have kept her from catching a cold from anyone. The long schedule of this event was a good test of her endurance so far.

June 9th was a visit to our neurologist again, the Best of the Best. He evaluated her muscle strength. He gave her a 5 on all but the front of her thighs. That was a 4 plus. We discussed reducing steroids from 20mg. He said to stay with the current dosage for 4 weeks and then go to 15mg. I brought up conversation about recovery odds. I had read that 60% of these cases relapse. **He expressed her odds of a full recovery as very good.**

June12th was another fundraising for her at a local golf course. I read a thank you letter to the crowd, acknowledging all their prayers and support. The place was packed. The band was great. The band learned the "Believe" tune for me. This was the one I sang at the fundraiser in the south. I could hardly finish it. This was a very emotional day. **She was able to dance and play golf**, something we only dreamed of a couple of months ago. Originally we thought it would be great if she could even do a ceremony of hitting the first ball. Spirits were high.

June 26th we went camping. She had tested the 3 stair approach, on the camper, a few weeks before and was thrilled to know **she could**

negotiate them. She felt she was getting back to normal events. Her strength was coming along. She enjoyed the weekend the way we used to. The pressure is lifting.

The weekend of July 30th she joined her group of women for their annual weekend of golf. Although she wasn't on par with her old form, she was well enough to go. On Saturday, July 31st, she got her very first hole-in-one. This is every golfer's dream. After the near death experience she survived, the mere thought of this boggles my mind. I have tears in my eyes as I am writing about it. She lived to enjoy one of the greatest moments in her life. It was surely a reward for her perseverance.

August 4th is another visit to the Best of the Best. We get a green light to **reduce steroids to 10mg**. He gave the ok to make this adjustment in 2 weeks. The muscles are still 5 except for the thigh at 4 plus. That one is going to take some work. We are to call him on August 25th **to go to**

7.5mg of steroids if she is tolerating the previous reduction well.

August 25th she called the doctor to report good health at 10mg of steroids. She did not get the doctor, but the assistant. She told the assistant she will go to 7.5mg dosage and to call her back if there is a problem with this.

September 21st she has to get some shots in her back for a previous ailment. The **Xarelto has to be stopped a few days before** because it is long lasting. She has to take shots of Lovanox for a few days in advance because it is fast acting and doesn't last in the blood stream. She can stop this medicine the day before. This will prevent bleeding problems during the procedure.

October 19th we had an agent from another health insurance company come to our house. This time we opted to this carrier because it was readily accepted in our southern home area.

Under the Medicare laws this company has all our needs covered.

October 20th again we visit the Best of the Best neurologist in our city. He hasn't changed his numbers on the muscles yet. He was surprised to learn that she went to 7.5mg of steroids. She told him of the discussion with the assistant. He said he never got word from the assistant. He will **continue steroids at 7.5mg per day** until we see our follow up doctor when we return to the south. His report said to go to 5mg per day after one month. We have to ask the new southern doctor if it is ok.

November 14th (one year since the first visit to the health clinic) we saw our new neurologist in our southern home area. We told her the northern doctor said we could go to 5mg per day after one month. That would be now. She prefers to **keep us on the same 7.5mg dose of steroids for four weeks longer**. We must be hitting a critical threshold. My wife wants to be done with them, but we must go with the doctor's guidance. Besides, some of her old aches and pains are returning with the reduction of steroids. 7.5mg must be a safer level. I did take notes at the visit. We were told to go to 5mg dosage after 4 more weeks. That would be just before Christmas. The previous doctors wanted to get off the very high doses, but seem comfortable at this level for now. She gave us a script to **get the Med-port removed** from her chest. We set the next visit for February 13th.

November 23rd we are back at our General Hospital in the south to get the Med-port removed. It is almost exactly **a year to the day** she entered the hospital and started this horrible journey. The Northern doctors told us to get it taken out at the facility where they put it in.

We got there early, like 7:20am. It is an hour drive. She weighed in at 137lbs. It was 10:20am when they finished all the questions and paperwork. We were escorted to a preparation room. I spent time in her room before they came for her at 10:35am.. I was told the procedure

took about 30 minutes. I went to the cafeteria for
a snack. I was called in from the waiting room
about 11:20am. She was bandaged up and would
be ready to leave after about and hour
observation time. Someone came in at 11:35am
to say she could leave at 12:09pm. We had to
laugh at the precise predicted time. It was
probably a type of humor designed to cheer up
the patient. I liked the approach. The nurse came
back at 11:55am to let her change into her street
clothes. We left at 12:09pm, believe it or not,
with a smile.

.....December 24th, there is a Christmas Eve
celebration at our recreation hall in the RV Park.
The members are going to parade their golf carts
through the park. They want my wife to lead the
parade in her hover scooter. They changed her to
the middle of the line up for her own protection.
They could keep a watch on her. She returned
early. The parade went on without her. Her little
scooter didn't have enough power to keep up
with the golf carts. This was a different Christmas
than the one a year earlier in ICU, by far.

January 20th, my wife and I discussed the previous instructions for the reduction of the steroid dosage. She says she has been taking 7.5mg. I reminded her of the November instructions of her new doctor. I had it in my notes. **She will start taking the 5mg dose tomorrow.** At this stage of our lives it is good to attend doctor visits together. Usually the one observing gets the message down. The one in the hot seat is not always focused.

February 13th we visited the neurologist we set up in the south. My wife finally passed all the muscle tests. She got a 5 rating on all muscle areas including the quadriceps. The doctor is looking forward to reducing the steroid dose to 2.5mg when she sees her in April.

February 20th we visited the primary doctor we use in the south. She wanted to eliminate the Xarelto. He wants to complete at least 1 year on it. Her Triglycerides were a bit high. He recommended diet adjustments for that. Another pill won't be necessary. It appears our doctoring visits are becoming a tolerable standard. Our future looks bright ahead.......for now.

IN CONCLUSION

In my opinion the best way to avoid NECROTIZING MYOPATHY due to STATIN DRUGS is to **stop taking the drug** at the first sign of pain, then, contact your doctor for advice and perhaps a prescription for a different brand of drug. A decision like **this is not life threatening at the moment**. You must have a frank discussion with your doctor. Trial and error, and blood tests, will guide you.

It may be necessary to take a "natural" route to lowering cholesterol.

We are still not finished with this unwanted journey. We have many follow up doctor visits ahead of us. They have indicated that the current medicines may go on for another year. The equipment we had to obtain is now stored in our basement; many various assists that she no longer requires.

We have asked three different lawyers to put

the original primary doctor on notice that this is unacceptable. The lawyers do not think there is sufficient evidence for a malpractice suit. We believe there is. I think these lawyers are in unfamiliar territory. This affliction is something they have rarely witnessed. Their letters of denial indicate they do not have sufficient medical advice to comfortably address the matter

We are settling into new routines that fit her needs. As we try to do the day-to-day things we are used to, we are interrupted by extra doctor visits and medicines we never needed before. We acquired a handicap sign to hang in our auto windshield. This gives her less walking in these busy areas. She is resorting to riding her bike in the neighborhood to strengthen her quadriceps. She has taken over control of her own medicine regiment, which is spelled out on the spreadsheet printed from our computer. **A copy of this list is especially helpful when visiting doctors.**

She seems to have reached a threshold in muscle development. The quadriceps muscles tire easily. Her weight has gone up about 10lbs since being discharged over ten months ago. The difficulty she faces is working that extra weight gain into more muscle matter. She is on a reduced dose of steroids, and wants to get off these extra medicines. The steroids are known to assist in muscle growth, so, it is probably a good thing to stay at this low dose for awhile. We only feel cautious of side effects, given all she has been through. Some of the puffy areas around her collar bone are receding. This was caused by the high dose of steroids. It is one of the side effects and an early stage of what they refer to as "Buffalo Hump".

Since the reduction of steroids to 5 mg, I notice she has a more difficult time going up stairs. The steroids must mask the fact that the muscles are taking a long time to reach their mature levels.

A couple of grab bars still remain in strategic places in the house. These are reassuring, but not used on a regular basis. However I do notice when she uses them. That is why they are still there.

The scooter we bought is not being used and now is in our way. I am entertaining the idea of selling it. Because of our age group, people we know are finding needs for some of our equipment for their loved ones. If I can find the right candidate I will give the scooter to them. It would be a way of "paying forward" for all the support we got along the way

Our feeling is there is little literature available to the average public for this problem. Medical journals can be too difficult to understand for many of us. We wanted our story to be told in order to help others cope with their own dealings with this affliction, or avoid it altogether.

As we have moved on, my wife and I are in constant discussions with others who have **corrected** their own **negative experiences with statin drugs**, some of them upon hearing of **our** plight. The problems of muscle pain are appearing to be more common than we imagined. The stories keep coming.

A friend told us her husband had such pain in the calves of his legs he could barely get out of bed. She took her husband off his cholesterol medicine and he is mobile again.

Another friend said he went through many brands of cholesterol medicine and still had the leg pain. He ached all over. His doctor finally agreed he was allergic to Cholesterol Medicine.

Another friend said she is taking the same cholesterol medicine as my wife did. She said she is going to monitor her results very carefully after knowing of my wife's plight.

Medicines are very necessary for so many of our sicknesses throughout our lives. They all seem to have an underlying danger. We read the warnings on the label, but we may not heed them as we should. This includes our doctors. It is up to us to respect the information we collect, and ask the proper questions. We can avoid a lot of problems associated with these medicine warnings, and lead a longer healthy life.

We can help control our own destiny.

We have to stay aware!

We have to keep the doctor aware.

We have to keep believing,

We have to keep moving on.

ABOUT THE AUTHOR

I should only say that I spent 80% to 90% of my time at my wife's side during her stay at the hospital. I looked out for her interests at every possible moment. My purpose was to fight for her when she couldn't. We are all able to understand pain. We have difficulty making good decisions when we are the one running scared. Someone has to think clearly and help make those choices.